T0344663

Ambulatory Urology and Urogynaecology

Ambulatory Urology and Urogynaecology

Edited by

Abhay Rane, OBE, MS, FRCS, FRCS(Urol)
Surrey and Sussex Healthcare NHS Trust
Redhill, Surrey, UK

Ajay Rane, OAM, MD, FRCOG, FRCS, FRANZCOG, CU, PhD, FICOG (Hon), FRCPI (Hon), GAICD, FACOG (Hon)
Department of Obstetrics and Gynaecology
James Cook University
Queensland, Australia

With co-editors

Jordan Durrant, MBBS, FRCS (Urol)
Department of Urology, East Surrey Hospital
Surrey, UK

Arjunan Tamilselvi, MBBS, DGO, FRCOG
Institute of Reproductive Medicine & Women's Health
Department of Urogynaecology, Madras Medical Mission Hospital
Chennai, India

Sandhya Gupta, MBBS, DGO, FRCOG, Dip Endoscopy
Department of Obstetrics and Gynaecology
The Townsville Hospital, Townsville, Australia

WILEY Blackwell

Registered Office(s)
John Wiley & Sons, Inc., 111 River Street, Hoboken, NJ 07030, USA
John Wiley & Sons Ltd, The Atrium, Southern Gate, Chichester, West Sussex, PO19 8SQ, UK

Editorial Office
9600 Garsington Road, Oxford, OX4 2DQ, UK

For details of our global editorial offices, customer services, and more information about Wiley products visit us at www.wiley.com.

Wiley also publishes its books in a variety of electronic formats and by print-on-demand. Some content that appears in standard print versions of this book may not be available in other formats.

Library of Congress Cataloging-in-Publication Data
Names: Rane, Abhay, editor. | Rane, Ajay, editor. |
    Durrant, Jordan, editor. | Tamilselvi, Arjunan, editor. | Gupta, Sandhya, editor.
Title: Ambulatory urology and urogynaecology / edited by Abhay Rane,
    Ajay Rane ; with co-editors, Jordan Durrant,
    Arjunan Tamilselvi, Sandhya Gupta.
Description: Hoboken, NJ : Wiley-Blackwell, [2021] | Includes
    bibliographical references and index.
Identifiers: LCCN 2020025492 (print) | LCCN 2020025493 (ebook) |
    ISBN 9781119052296 (hardback) | ISBN 9781119052272 (adobe pdf) | ISBN 9781119052265 (epub)
Subjects: MESH: Urologic Diseases–surgery | Urologic Surgical Procedures |
    Ambulatory Surgical Procedures
Classification: LCC RD571 (print) | LCC RD571 (ebook) | NLM WJ 168 |
    DDC 617.4/610597–dc23
LC record available at https://lccn.loc.gov/2020025492
LC ebook record available at https://lccn.loc.gov/2020025493

Cover Design: Wiley
Cover Images: © SEBASTIAN KAULITZKI /SCIENCE PHOTO LIBRARY/ Getty Images,
© SCIEPRO/Getty Images

Set in 9.5/12.5pt STIXTwoText by SPi Global, Pondicherry, India
Printed and bound by CPI Group (UK) Ltd, Croydon, CR0 4YY

10 9 8 7 6 5 4 3 2 1

This book is dedicated to our parents, Murali and Snehalata, who gave us everything.

Contents

List of Contributors

Editors

Abhay Rane OBE, MS, FRCS, FRCS(Urol)
Professor of Urology
Surrey and Sussex Healthcare NHS Trust
Redhill, Surrey, UK

**Ajay Rane, OAM, MD, FRCOG, FRCS,
FRANZCOG, CU, PhD, FICOG (Hon),
FRCPI (Hon), GAICD, FACOG (Hon)**
Consultant Urogynaecologist
Department of Obstetrics and
Gynaecology
James Cook University
Queensland, Australia

Contributors

**Hussain Alnajjar, MBBS ChM (Urol),
FEBU FRCS (Urol)**
Department of Urology and Andrology
University College London Hospitals
NHS Trust
United Kingdom

G. Willy Davila, MD, FACOG (FPMRS)
Director of Women and Children's Services
Holy Cross Medical Group
Dorothy Mangurian Comprehensive
Women's Center
Fort Lauderdale
FL, USA

Jordan Durrant, MBBS, FRCS (Urol)
Department of Urology
East Surrey Hospital
Surrey; Sussex Healthcare
NHS Trust
United Kingdom

**Sandhya Gupta, MBBS, DGO, FRCOG, Dip
Endoscopy**
Specialist, Department of Obstetrics
and Gynaecology
The Townsville Hospital
Townsville, Australia

**Khaled M.K. Ismail, MBBCh,
MSc, MD, PhD**
Professor
Department of Gynecology and
Obstetrics
Faculty of Medicine in Pilsen
University Hospital Pilsen
Charles University
Czech Republic

**Jay Iyer, MBBS, MD, DNB, FRCOG,
FRANZCOG**
Specialist, Department of Obstetrics
and Gynaecology
The Townsville Hospital
Townsville, Australia

Vladimir Kalis, MD, PhD
Associate Professor
Department of Gynecology and
Obstetrics
Faculty of Medicine in Pilsen
University Hospital Pilsen
Charles University
Czech Republic

Rasha Kamel, MBBCh, MSc, MD
Professor
Maternal-Fetal Medicine Unit
Department of Obstetrics and
Gynecology
Cairo University
Egypt

Mugdha Kulkarni, MBBS, FRANZCOG
Urogynaecology Fellow
Monash Health
Melbourne, Australia

Tharani Mahesan, MBBS, BSc, MRCS
Department of Urology
East Surrey Hospital
Surrey and Sussex Healthcare
NHS Trust
United Kingdom

Tharani Nitkunan, BSc Hons, MBBS, PhD, FRCS (Urol)
Department of Urology
Epsom and St Helier University
Hospitals NHS Trust
United Kingdom

Aakash Pai, BSc, MBBS, FRCS (Urol)
Department of Urology
Northampton General Hospital
NHS Trust
United Kingdom

Ashiv Patel, MBBS
Department of Urology
East Surrey Hospital
Surrey and Sussex Healthcare NHS Trust
United Kingdom

Benjamin Patel, BA, BM BCh
Department of Urology
East Surrey Hospital
Surrey and Sussex Healthcare NHS Trust
United Kingdom

Ben Pullar, MBBS, BSc, FRCS (Urol)
Department of Urology
The Lister Hospital
Stevenage, United Kingdom

Karen Randhawa, MBChB, MFST(Ed), FRCS (Urol)
Department of Urology and Andrology
University College London
Hospitals NHS Trust
United Kingdom

Angie Rantell, PhD, RCN, ALNP
Lead Nurse, Urogynaecology/Nurse
Cystoscopist
King's College Hospital
London, United Kingdom

Dudley Robinson, MD, FRCOG
Department of Urogynaecology
King's College Hospital
London, United Kingdom

Anna Rosamilia, MBBS, FRANZCOG, CU, PhD
Urogynaecologist and Head of Pelvic
Floor Unit
Monash Health
Melbourne, Australia

Mark Salmon, MBBS, FRCA, DipIMC
Department of Anaesthesia
East Surrey Hospital
Surrey and Sussex Healthcare
NHS Trust
United Kingdom

Marcella Zanzarini Sanson
Department of Obstetrics and
Gynecology
Medical School of Ribeirão Preto
University of São Paulo
Brazil

Tanvir Singh, MB, BS, MS – OBGyn,
Bachelor Endoscopy – MIS
Consultant
Department of Obstetrics and
Gynaecology
Tanvir Hospital
Hyderabad, India

Arjunan Tamilselvi, MBBS, DGO, FRCOG
Consultant Urogynaecologist and
Pelvic Surgeon
Department of Urogynaecology
Institute of Reproductive Medicine &
Women's Health
Madras Medical Mission Hospital
Chennai, India

David Thurtle, BMBS, BMedSci, MRCS
Department of Urology
University of Cambridge and North
West Anglia NHS Foundation Trust
United Kingdom

Karan Wadhwa, PhD (Cantab),
FRCS (Urol)
Department of Urology
Mid and South Essex NHS Trust
United Kingdom

Sylvia Yan, MBChB, MRCS
Department of Urology
Epsom and St Helier University
Hospitals NHS Trust
United Kingdom

Section I

Basic Principles of an Ambulatory Service

1

Principles of an Ambulatory Surgery Service

Mark Salmon and Benjamin Patel

According to the International Association for Ambulatory Surgery (IAAS), ambulatory surgery should be defined as 'an operation/procedure, excluding an office or outpatient operation/procedure, where the patient is discharged on the same working day.' The origins of ambulatory surgery can be traced back to the pioneering work of James Nicholl at the Glasgow Royal Hospital who reported 8988 paediatric day- case procedures between 1899 and 1908. Despite initial scepticism from the surgical profession, there has been a rapid expansion in the complexity and amount of ambulatory surgery in recent years: between 1989 and 2003 the percentage of elective surgery undertaken as day case in the UK increased from 15 to 70%. Many health services have set targets for the percentage of elective surgeries to be done as day-case procedures, and in the UK this target is set at 75%.

The rise of ambulatory surgery has been driven by technological advances that reduce the need for overnight hospital stays, enhanced recovery programmes that advocate early mobilisation, and the need for economic efficiency. With growing interest in ambulatory surgery, multiple associations have been formed promoting education, quality standards, and research in the field.

Infrastructure

Ambulatory care is delivered in various environments, including

- Free-standing self-contained units
- Integrated self-contained units
- Integrated non-self-contained units

Ambulatory Urology and Urogynaecology, First Edition. Edited by Abhay Rane and Ajay Rane.
© 2021 John Wiley & Sons Ltd. Published 2021 by John Wiley & Sons Ltd.

Free-standing units, separate to inpatient units, are common in the United States, increasing in number from 67 in 1976 to over 4000 in 2004 (IAAS: day surgery). They may be multidisciplinary, serving a larger market, or uni-disciplinary. Potential benefits include cost-effectiveness and efficiency because it is easier to generate a streamlined care pathway and to encourage teamwork amongst healthcare professionals. Furthermore, they may have lower rates of hospital-acquired infection. The disadvantage is that they are remote from a comprehensive medical facility with a full range of specialties including intensive care, meaning that there will occasionally be a need for outsourcing and transfer of patients. The need for low-risk patients ultimately encourages stricter patient selection, self-limiting the service. Most unplanned overnight admissions after ambulatory surgery are due to bleeding and longer-than-expected procedure length, with urological and gynaecological surgery accounting for a particularly high proportion of bleeding patients (Vaghadia 1998).

Integrated self-contained ambulatory units are located on a hospital site with their own dedicated theatres and personnel. They are generally seen as the ideal model for ambulatory surgery, benefiting from the comprehensive range of medical services provided by that hospital, whilst also specialising in providing a streamlined ambulatory service with one dedicated team well trained in ambulatory surgical care.

Integrated non-self-contained ambulatory units vary significantly in set-up: some may not have dedicated theatres or personnel. This makes the system inefficient, because there is a chance that low-risk day-case procedures may be cancelled, a streamlined patient pathway is often lacking, and unintended overnight stays arise due to difficulties ensuring safe discharge. However, if there is a dedicated ambulatory ward and theatres, this environment does have some benefits; it is easily expandable, meaning that as new procedures are transferred to day surgery, the same infrastructure can be used with appropriate retraining of staff.

Pre-operative Assessment

Once the decision to operate has been established and the intended procedure is planned as a day case, a dedicated pre-assessment team, generally made up of trained nurses, should comprehensively assess the patient. This assessment should ideally take place in the same unit in which the procedure will take place but can be undertaken remotely via telephone or computer. It should happen far enough in advance so that patients' co-morbidities, medications, and social factors can be optimised preoperatively.

The pre-operative assessment begins with gathering information about health, medications, and social circumstance. The health assessment is generally history-based and most commonly involves a questionnaire with basic screening questions and more detailed history where appropriate. Pre-operative examination and investigations including blood tests, ECG, and X-rays are less useful in most patients. A decision is then made regarding whether the patient is suitable for day surgery. Modern ambulatory units have moved away from a specific set of contraindications and instead assess patient suitability individually according to the combination of physiological status, social circumstance and intended procedure.

Social Selection Criteria

Several social factors must be considered before ambulatory surgery. Patients or carers must be able to understand the nature of the procedure, and be willing to adhere to the peri-operative instructions. Patients must have appropriate support at home; in general, they need to be discharged into the care of a responsible adult for 24 hours after the operation, although this is probably excessive for some minor operations. Additionally, a generally accepted rule is that they must live within one hour's travel time to the surgical unit. In those living remote from ambulatory unit, the option of an overnight local lodging can be discussed, instead of overnight hospital admission.

Physical Selection Criteria

There are multiple factors that reduce the suitability of patients for day surgery and must be assessed in detail prior to surgery (Fong 2014). Identifying high-risk patients can help facilitate a multidisciplinary strategy to optimise their pre-operative condition, anticipate intraoperative challenges, and plan postoperative disposition (Walsh 2018). Although a comprehensive review of these is beyond the scope of this chapter, we will mention a few notable parameters.

Age should not independently decide whether a patient is suitable. In one study, elderly patients did not have worse outcomes than younger patients (Chung 1999), although in another, advanced age was associated with greater rates of readmission (Whippey 2013). Ambulatory surgery may actually confer some benefits to the elderly population, having been shown to reduce rates of post-operative cognitive dysfunction (Rasmussen 2015).

The American Society of Anaesthesiologists grading system (ASA grade) is used to evaluate a patient's physical state before surgery and classifies patients into

6 categories. Grade 1 being a normal healthy patient and grade 5 being moribund patient. The ASA grade is not a particularly useful measure of suitability for day surgery. An ASA 3 patient does not experience greater complication rates when compared to an ASA 1 or 2 in the medium to late post-operative period (Ansell 2004). Some ASA 4 patients may also be suitable for procedures undertaken using local or regional anaesthesia.

Suitability of obese patients is a controversial area, a body mass index (BMI) of up to 40 being acceptable for the majority of procedures and many anaesthetists would accept higher BMIs (Atkins 2002). Complication rates do appear to be higher in the extremely obese group (BMI > 50 kg/m^2), although readmission rates are not significantly greater (Joshi 2013).

With regards to chronic medical conditions, a general rule is that stable patients are fit for ambulatory surgery. Chronic obstructive pulmonary disease (COPD) is not a contraindication for ambulatory surgery. Asymptomatic patients have a low risk of post-operative complications, but those who have been symptomatic within a month of the proposed surgery may need to have their procedure postponed (Warner 1996). Smokers should be encouraged to stop smoking, as even short-term cessation pre-operatively has been demonstrated to reduce complications (Myles 2002). Patients with obstructive sleep apnoea should have good control of symptoms and be established on nasal continuous positive airway pressure pre-operatively and during the post-operative period.

Cardiovascular status should also be assessed pre-operatively. Patients with hypertension should have their blood pressure reasonably controlled. The majority of those with ischaemic heart disease will be suitable, except for those with unstable or severe angina and those who have experienced recent myocardial infarction. Additionally, ambulatory surgery is generally not undertaken within a year of drug-eluting stent placement (Wijeysundera 2012). Diabetes mellitus does not itself preclude a patient from day surgery; in fact, day surgery reduces disruption to normal routine. However, patients should ideally be screened for other co-morbidities including cardiovascular and renal dysfunction. Patients with end-stage renal failure may be appropriate for minor ambulatory procedures undertaken under local or regional anaesthesia but, given their poor physiological state and the practical issues with regards to dialysis, major ambulatory operations are generally contraindicated.

Preparation for Surgery

Once the patient has been adequately assessed and deemed suitable for ambulatory surgery, the clinical team will start to prepare. This will involve completion of any further anaesthetic investigations and surgical diagnostics. Consent should be obtained with explanation and post-operative plan discussed.

The patient must be given appropriate information regarding the perioperative period. This will include an overview of fasting requirements, medications that need to be taken, and information pertaining to personal hygiene. In addition, simple information about location and timings should be provided. Finally, the patient and carer/responsible adult should be given information on whom to contact for queries or help with post-operative complications.

Anaesthesia

Pre-operatively, a full anaesthetic assessment should be performed, including previous anaesthetic history, post-operative nausea and vomiting (PONV) risk, and an airway assessment. PONV a common complication of anaesthesia, occurs most often in females, those with a similar past history, those with motion sickness, nonsmokers, and those requiring post-operative opioids (Apfel 1999). Pre-operative assessment should aim to identify risk factors for difficult pain control allowing for individualised perioperative analgesia planning.

Most current anaesthetic agents convey predictable and rapid recovery. Desflurane-based anaesthetic has been reported to have the most predictable emergence from anaesthesia (Dexter 2011; Watchel 2011), although desflurane and sevoflurane-based anaesthesia appear to provide equal numbers of patients eligible for fast-tracking (White 2009). Propofol is frequently used for induction and maintenance of ambulatory anaesthesia, due to rapid metabolism and emergence, few side-effects, and low rates of PONV.

Depth of anaesthesia monitors, such as Bi-spectral Index (BIS), facilitate drug titration and have been shown to reduce drug consumption, reduce PONV (Liu 2004), and reduce rates of post-operative cognitive dysfunction in elderly patients (Chan 2013).

Post-operative pain will vary according to patient factors as well as the specifics of the surgical procedure and anaesthesia used. Utilising minimally invasive surgical techniques and regional anaesthesia are obvious ways to reduce pain. Regional anaesthetic techniques such as peripheral nerve blockade or neuraxial blockade, can mitigate the side effects of general anaesthesia such as PONV and aspiration pneumonia and may accelerate recovery by facilitating early analgesia (Moore 2013) and reducing opioid requirement. For neuraxial blocks, drug selection and dosing must be carefully considered so that prolonged effects do not delay discharge.

A number of antiemetics have been investigated and compared for efficacy. The 5HT3 antagonists such as ondansetron have good efficacy, especially when used in combination with dexamethasone. These should be started before the end of anaesthesia (Tang 1998) and continued in the community if necessary. Side effects should be evaluated when choosing an agent. Dexamethasone should be avoided in patients with lymphoma because of risk of tumour lysis syndrome. Ondansetron should be avoided in patients with, or at risk of long QT.

Early Recovery: Emergence from Anaesthesia

Early recovery commences from the discontinuation of anaesthetic agents, allowing the patient to emerge from anaesthesia, recover airway reflexes and resume motor activity. Classically, this occurs in the post-anaesthesia care unit (PACU), before stepping down to the day-surgery unit (DSU). The modified Aldrete scoring system can be used for determining when patients are fit for discharge from PACU (Aldrete 1995).

There is a growing trend towards 'fast-track' of patients directly from the operating theatre to the DSU, bypassing PACU. This is (i) safe as many patients achieve step-down criteria from PACU as soon as they arrive, and (ii) economically efficient as PACU is more labour intensive. Complication rates in PACU are low, with one group demonstrating rates of 8%, of which only 0.7% were respiratory or circulatory (Duncan 1992).

One group achieved fast-track rates of over 80% in simple orthopaedic procedures, with patients being successfully discharged home earlier (Duncan 2001). Fast-track is more achievable with desflurane and sevoflurane-based anaesthesia (Song 1998) and with BIS, ensuring minimum necessary anaesthesia and quicker recovery (Song 1997).

The modified Aldrete scoring system is limited in deciding whether patients are fit for fast-track as it does not consider pain, nausea, or vomiting which are generally addressed in PACU. White's criteria (White 1999), or the WAKE score (2011) are more appropriate. Ultimately, patient safety should always be maintained and a clinical judgement should be made as to whether fast-track is appropriate.

Achieving adequate pain relief is an important factor for patient satisfaction and should be managed with objective methods of pain evaluation and evidence-based protocols for pain control. Utilisation of ibuprofen and celecoxib have been demonstrated to improve recovery (White 2011), probably because they are associated with lower opioid requirements and reduction of oedema. Units have developed protocols with routine use of multimodal analgesia, including non-steroidal anti-inflammatory drugs (NSAID), local anaesthetic techniques, and opioids as necessary. These protocols and methods have demonstrated improved post-operative pain control and patient satisfaction (Elvir-Lazo 2010).

Intermediate Recovery: Discharge Criteria

There is an increasing pressure for rapid discharge of patients. However, this must be balanced with the risks associated with premature discharge, including readmission, complications, and legal consequences. Several scoring systems exist, guiding clinicians about safe discharge. The Post Anaesthesia Discharge Scoring System (PADS) (Chung 1995) is one utilised example and includes observations, patient orientation, bleeding, and post-operative symptoms including pain and nausea. Post-operative voiding and tolerance of oral intake are also included in this scoring system.

The type of anaesthesia and surgery can be a determinant of post-operative voiding function. Specific to pelvic-floor procedures is the effect of anaesthesia on bladder function. The insertion of the mid-urethral sling has been performed under both regional and local anaesthetic, with regional anaesthesia having been found to increase the rates of post-operative urinary retention (Adjusted OR = 4.4, 95% CI 1.9, 10.2) (Wohlrab 2009), a factor that could influence length of stay. A systematic review looking at the effect of anaesthesia on bladder function, found the dose of intrathecal local anaesthetic used with regional anaesthetic, as well as the potency of the anaesthetic used, to correlate with the duration of bladder dysfunction (Choi 2012). Encouragingly, a retrospective review of 119 patients who were discharged the same day as undergoing outpatient tension-free vaginal tape (TVT) surgeries found no significant difference in the need for catheterization among patients who received spinal anaesthesia compared to those who received general or local anaesthetic with sedation (Barron 2006).

Voiding before discharge has been a core concept in ambulatory surgery, because of the concern that patients may develop urinary retention, bladder atony, and subsequently renal complications. However, there is good evidence (Pavlin 1999) that patients at low risk of urinary retention can be discharged without needing to void, but with clear instructions to seek medical attention if unable to void within eight hours of discharge. On the other hand, the literature and opinions are mixed regarding patients at high risk of retention. Guidelines support that those who have not voided within three hours post-operatively should receive bladder scanning; if >600mls is present, then they will need catheterisation with trial without catheter (TWOC) in the community (Pavlin 1999).

Tolerance of oral fluids was also previously mandated before discharge. However, several studies have proven that this does not improve outcomes and may even worsen rates of nausea and vomiting (Jin 1998, Kearney 1998), making this a historic requirement.

Once discharge criteria have been met, patients should be supplied with adequate analgesia and clear instructions to take it regularly to prevent breakthrough pain. Prepackaged medication is convenient, prevents delays, and eliminates the need for a patient or carer to visit the pharmacy. Patients should be given clear verbal and written instructions on what they should and should not do, alongside contact details in case of emergency or concerns about symptoms or complications. Patients should be discharged with a responsible adult to accompany them, and those who have had a general anaesthetic should be advised to avoid alcohol and driving for 24 hours.

Late Recovery: Care After Discharge

Patients are discharged from ambulatory surgery once their baseline physiological states have returned. Although major complications and morbidity are rare (Warner 1993), residual symptoms and side effects are not uncommon. Patients need to be followed up in the community. This can happen through telephone consultations (Kamming 2004), GP/nursing follow-up, outpatient clinics or 'mhealth apps,' on smartphones (Hwa 2013, Armstrong 2014). A dedicated contact phone number or routine follow-up call the next day, may help avoid unscheduled emergency or general practitioner visits after discharge. Telephone follow up has reported high satisfaction rates (>90%) with all women preferring it to an office visit (Schimpf 2016). Ambulatory centres should consider this as a routine part of their postprocedure care. Follow-up should consider pain, nausea, bleeding, oral intake, voiding, bowel function, fever, sore throat, disorientation, and psychological status.

Setting Up an Ambulatory Centre

Planning a new ambulatory unit is a major undertaking. A board team, consisting of at least a surgeon, anaesthetist, nurse, and project manager should be set up. Market research must be performed, considering demand and financial viability. Local health authorities and regulatory bodies must be involved. The location must be identified taking into account transport links, and infrastructure must be decided upon.

Staff must be recruited and appropriately trained. Nurses must be educated in pre-operative triage/assessment and be trained in assessing patients postoperatively for discharge using standardised protocols. They should be able to engage the patient and family in the process of ambulatory surgery to ensure compliance and success. Anaesthetic teams must be trained in appropriate techniques for day surgery. Surgical teams must stay up to date with guidelines, such as the British Association of Day Surgery (BADS) directory, which makes recommendations on which procedures are appropriate in the ambulatory setting. All groups should demonstrate competency in dealing with emergency scenarios.

An ambulatory surgical checklist should be developed and tailored to different specialities. Staff should be trained in communication skills. The 'Situation-Background-Assessment-Recommendation (SBAR)' tool is a useful framework. Formal training in teamwork should ideally be given, generating a patient-centred culture of safety. Systems should be established to deal with unprofessional behaviour, mistakes, and complaints. An audit and quality improvement team must be set up. Staff must be trained in hand hygiene and infection control.

The design of the unit is central to its success. The capacity must be determined, including theatre number and bed number. From this, an estimate of size can be extrapolated. The board team and architect must decide on build type, storage, and sterilisation facilities. They then must consider which 'model' to follow. The 'racetrack' model has a uni-directional flow path, meaning that pre- and post-operative patients are not mixed and there is no congestion of flow. The disadvantage of this model is that more space is required to house pre- and post-operative patients in separate areas and at certain times of the day, there will be unused space. The 'non-racetrack' model conversely does mix patients, economising on space, but possibly at the detriment of quality.

Following this, members of the board team need to consider space for reception, patient's changing rooms, toilets, consulting rooms, staff common rooms and catering facilities. Medical gas supply must be incorporated into the design. Hardware such as trolleys, operating tables, beds, blood fridges, and emergency trolleys must be thought out. Operating theatres must be designed and anaesthetic equipment taken into account.

Following the design, a business plan should be constructed, including the capital costs, income, and expenditure over the next five years. This will need to be presented to investors or local funding panels

Economics of Ambulatory Surgery

The economic benefits of ambulatory surgery are a major drive for uptake. A number of studies have demonstrated the cost-effectiveness of various procedures when performed in the outpatient versus inpatient setting (Hollingsworth 2012). In 1990, the UK's Audit Commission suggested that if all health authorities in England and Wales performed day surgery consistently for 20 common procedures, an additional 186 000 patients could be treated each year without increased costs. This led to the England's Department of Health recommendation that 75% of all elective surgery be undertaken as day-case procedures (Alan Milburn NHS plan 2002). The UK Department of Health's reference costs for 2013–2014 calculated that the average day-case cost was £698 compared to £3375 for elective inpatient cases (reference costs 2013–2014).

These economic benefits stem from shorter hospital stays, with reduced waiting lists and higher patient turnover; fixed scheduling with reduced cancellations; staff reductions with lower overnight capacity; reduced operating times and lower costs associated with post-operative care (Aboutarabi 2014). Furthermore, patients benefit from reduced disruption from normal routine and quicker recovery back to work.

Various strategies have been proposed to economise even further within ambulatory surgery. Nerve blocks for reduction of pain, fast-tracking, and modifying the type and amount of anaesthesia have all been investigated in detail. Future innovations in terms of surgical technology and technique, anaesthesia and post-operative monitoring including the use of telemedicine will likely further the scope and economic efficiency of ambulatory surgery.

Complication Rates

Transfer to an acute care facility or hospitalisation after discharge is often used as a marker of the complication rate for day-care surgery. Outpatient gynaecological and urogynaecology procedures have been successfully performed with very few patients (1.6%) requiring inpatient treatment within 72 hours (Kannan 2008). Similar results have been replicated in numerous studies of urology patients.

A multicentre quality improvement project performed in the USA found that 12% of patients undergoing other ambulatory surgery required hospital transfer and 10% required hospitalisation or an emergency room attendance within 48 hours of discharge from the day-care unit (Davis 2019).

Conclusion

Redistributing surgical procedures from the inpatient setting to ambulatory centres can be done without impacting quality. Ambulatory surgery confers substantial advantage and will continue to increase in popularity, in line with economic pressures. Re-evaluation and improvement are central to its success and units should routinely audit their cases and outcomes, along with the incorporation of novel techniques and innovations.

Further Reading

Aboutorabi, A., Ghiasipour, M., Rezapour, A. et al. (2014 Spring). A cost-minimization analysis of day-care versus in-patient surgery for five most common general surgical procedures. *Journal of Health Policy and Sustainable Health*. 1 (2): 33–36.

Aldrete, J.A. (1995 Feb). The post-anesthesia recovery score revisited. *J Clin Anesth*. 7 (1): 89–91.

Ansell, G.L. and Montgomery, J.E. (2004 Jan). Outcome of ASA III patients undergoing day case surgery. *Br J Anaesth*. 92 (1): 71–74.

Apfel, C.C., Läärä, E., Koivuranta, M. et al. (1999 Sep). A simplified risk score for predicting postoperative nausea and vomiting: conclusions from cross-validations between two centers. *Anesthesiology*. 91 (3): 693–700.

Armstrong, K.A., Semple, J.L., and Coyte, P.C. (2014 Sep 22). Replacing ambulatory surgical follow-up visits with mobile app home monitoring: modeling cost-effective scenarios. *J Med Internet Res.* 16 (9): e213.

Atkins, M., White, J., and Ahmed, K. (2002). Day surgery and body mass index: results of a national survey. *Anaesthesia.* 57 (2): 169–182.

Barron, K.I., Savageau, J.A., Young, S.B. et al. (2006). Prediction of successful voiding immediately after outpatient mid-urethral sling. *Int Urogynecol J Pelvic Floor Dysfunct.* 17 (6): 570–575. https://doi.org/10.1007/s00192-005-0064-8.

Chan, M.T.V., Cheng, B.C.P., Lee, T.M.C. et al. (2013 Jan). BIS-guided anesthesia decreases postoperative delirium and cognitive decline. *J Neurosurg Anesthesiol.* 25 (1): 33.

Choi, S., Mahon, P., and Awad, I.T. (2012). Neuraxial anesthesia and bladder dysfunction in the perioperative period: a systematic review [published correction appears in Can J Anaesth. 2017 Dec 18]. *Can J Anaesth.* 59 (7): 681–703.

Chung, F., Chan, V.W., and Ong, D. (1995 Sep). A post-anesthetic discharge scoring system for home readiness after ambulatory surgery. *J Clin Anesth.* 7 (6): 500–506.

Chung, F., Mezei, G., and Tong, D. (1999 Apr 1). Adverse events in ambulatory surgery. A comparison between elderly and younger patients. *Can J Anaesth.* 46 (4): 309.

Davis, K.K., Mahishi, V., Singal, R. et al. (2019). Quality Improvement in Ambulatory Surgery Centers: A Major National Effort Aimed at Reducing Infections and Other Surgical Complications. *J Clin Med Res.* 11 (1): 7–14.

Dexter, F., Bayman, E.O., and Epstein, R.H. (2010 Feb 1). Statistical modeling of average and variability of time to extubation for meta-analysis comparing desflurane to sevoflurane. *Anesth Analg.* 110 (2): 570–580.

Duncan, P.G., Cohen, M.M., Tweed, W.A. et al. (1992 May 1). The Canadian four-centre study of anaesthetic outcomes: III. Are anaesthetic complications predictable in day surgical practice? *Can J Anaesth.* 39 (5): 440.

Duncan, P.G., Shandro, J., Bachand, R., and Ainsworth, L. (2001 Aug). A pilot study of recovery room bypass ("fast-track protocol") in a community hospital. *Can J Anaesth.* 48 (7): 630–636.

Elvir-Lazo, O.L. and White, P.F. (2010). Postoperative pain management after ambulatory surgery: role of multimodal analgesia. *Anesthesiol Clin.* 28 (2): 217–224.

Fong, R. and Sweitzer, B.J. (2014 Dec 1). Preoperative optimization of patients undergoing ambulatory surgery. *Curr Anesthesiol Rep.* 4 (4): 303–315.

Hollingsworth, J.M., Saigal, C.S., Lai, J.C. et al. (2012). Surgical quality among Medicare beneficiaries undergoing outpatient urological surgery. *J Urol.* 188 (4): 1274–1278.

Hwa, K. and Wren, S.M. (2013 Sep). Telehealth follow-up in lieu of postoperative clinic visit for ambulatory surgery: results of a pilot program. *JAMA Surg.* 148 (9): 823–827.

Jin, F., Norris, A., Chung, F., and Ganeshram, T. (1998 Aug). Should adult patients drink fluids before discharge from ambulatory surgery? *Anesth Analg.* 87 (2): 306–311.

Joshi, G.P., Ahmad, S., Riad, W. et al. (2013 Nov). Selection of obese patients undergoing ambulatory surgery: a systematic review of the literature. *Anesth Analg.* 117 (5): 1082–1091.

Kamming, D., Chung, F., Williams, D. et al. (2004 Jun). Pain management in ambulatory surgery. *J Perianesthesia Nurs Off J Am Soc PeriAnesthesia Nurses.* 19 (3): 174–182.

Kannan, K., Kasper, A., Balakrishnan, S., and Rane, A. (2008 Winter). Ambulatory gynaecology and urogynaecology procedures: a viable option? *Australian and New Zealand Continence Journal.* 14 (2): 38–42.

Kearney, R., Mack, C., and Entwistle, L. (1998). Withholding oral fluids from children undergoing day surgery reduces vomiting. *Paediatr Anaesth.* 8 (4): 331–336.

Liu, S.S. (2004 Aug). Effects of Bispectral Index monitoring on ambulatory anesthesia: a meta-analysis of randomized controlled trials and a cost analysis. *Anesthesiology.* 101 (2): 311–315.

Moore, J.G., Ross, S.M., and Williams, B.A. (2013 Dec). Regional anesthesia and ambulatory surgery. *Curr Opin Anaesthesiol.* 26 (6): 652–660.

Myles, P.S., Iacono, G.A., Hunt, J.O. et al. (2002 Oct). Risk of respiratory complications and wound infection in patients undergoing ambulatory surgery: smokers versus nonsmokers. *Anesthesiology.* 97 (4): 842–847.

Pavlin, D.J., Pavlin, E.G., Fitzgibbon, D.R. et al. (1999 Jul). Management of bladder function after outpatient surgery. *Anesthesiology.* 91 (1): 42–50.

Pavlin, D.J., Pavlin, E.G., Gunn, H.C. et al. (1999 Jul). Voiding in patients managed with or without ultrasound monitoring of bladder volume after outpatient surgery. *Anesth Analg.* 89 (1): 90–97.

Rasmussen, L.S. and Steinmetz, J. (2015 Dec). Ambulatory anaesthesia and cognitive dysfunction. *Curr Opin Anaesthesiol.* 28 (6): 631–635.

Schimpf, M.O., Fenner, D.E., Smith, T.M. et al. (2016). Patient satisfaction with nurse-led telephone follow-up in an ambulatory setting. *Female Pelvic Med Reconstr Surg.* 22 (6): 430–432.

Song, D., Joshi, G.P., and White, P.F. (1997 Oct). Titration of volatile anesthetics using bispectral index facilitates recovery after ambulatory anesthesia. *Anesthesiology.* 87 (4): 842–848.

Song, D., Joshi, G.P., and White, P.F. (1998 Feb). Fast-track eligibility after ambulatory anesthesia: a comparison of desflurane, sevoflurane, and propofol. *Anesth Analg.* 86 (2): 267–273.

Vaghadia, H., Scheepers, L., and Merrick, P.M. (1998 Nov). Readmission for bleeding after outpatient surgery. *Can J Anaesth.* 45 (11): 1079–1083.

Wachtel, R.E., Dexter, F., Epstein, R.H., and Ledolter, J. (2011 Aug). Meta-analysis of desflurane and propofol average times and variability in times to extubation and following commands. *Can J Anaesth.* 58 (8): 714–724.

Walsh, M.T. (2018). Improving outcomes in ambulatory anesthesia by identifying high risk patients. *Curr Opin Anaesthesiol.* 31 (6): 659–666.

Warner, D.O., Warner, M.A., Barnes, R.D. et al. (1996 Sep). Perioperative respiratory complications in patients with asthma. *Anesthesiology.* 85 (3): 460–467.

Warner, M.A., Shields, S.E., and Chute, C.G. (1993 Sep 22). Major morbidity and mortality within 1 month of ambulatory surgery and anesthesia. *JAMA.* 270 (12): 1437–1441.

Whippey, A., Kostandoff, G., Paul, J. et al. (2013 Jul 1). Predictors of unanticipated admission following ambulatory surgery: a retrospective case-control study. *Can J Anesth* 60 (7): 675–683.

White, P.F. and Song, D. (1999 May). New criteria for fast-tracking after outpatient anesthesia: a comparison with the modified Aldrete's scoring system. *Anesth Analg.* 88 (5): 1069–1072.

White, P.F., Tang, J., Wender, R.H. et al. (2009 Aug). Desflurane versus sevoflurane for maintenance of outpatient anesthesia: the effect on early versus late recovery and perioperative coughing. *Anesth Analg.* 109 (2): 387–393.

Wijeysundera, D.N., Wijeysundera, H.C., Yun, L. et al. (2012 Sep 11). Risk of elective major noncardiac surgery after coronary stent insertion: a population-based study. *Circulation.* 126 (11): 1355–1362.

Williams, B.A. and Kentor, M.L. (2011). The WAKE© score: patient-centered ambulatory anesthesia and fast-tracking outcomes criteria. *Int Anesthesiol Clin.* 49 (3): 33–43.

Section II

Ambulatory Urogynaecology

2

Introduction and Epidemiology of Pelvic Floor Dysfunction

Jay Iyer and Ajay Rane

Introduction

The pelvic floor consists of the muscles, ligaments, and connective tissue that constitute the pelvic organ supports. The pelvic organs include the bladder, uterus and cervix, vagina, rectum and bowel. The supporting pelvic floor not only prevents the descent of these organs, but also maintains their anatomical position and helps in their normal function. Pelvic floor dysfunction (PFD) is a group of disorders that affects these various structures and can therefore lead to bladder and/or bowel dysfunction.The condition cannot only affect daily activities, sexual function, and exercise, but it can also impact negatively on one's emotional and psychological state. The presence of pelvic floor dysfunction can have a detrimental impact on body image and sexuality. Diagnosis is often delayed because most women are embarrassed to discuss their condition.

Types of Pelvic Floor Dysfunction

Pelvic Organ Prolapse (POP)

The International Continence Society (ICS) defines prolapse as the descent of one or more of the anterior vaginal wall, the posterior vaginal wall, and the apex or the vault of the vagina. Symptoms generally include difficulty in emptying the bladder or rectum, urinary or faecal incontinence, pelvic pressure, vaginal bulge and/or sexual dysfunction.

Ambulatory Urology and Urogynaecology, First Edition. Edited by Abhay Rane and Ajay Rane.
© 2021 John Wiley & Sons Ltd. Published 2021 by John Wiley & Sons Ltd.

Urinary Incontinence

ICS defines urinary incontinence (UI) as the involuntary loss of urine. The most common recognised subtypes of UI are stress urinary incontinence (SUI), urge urinary incontinence (UUI), and mixed urinary incontinence (MUI). Overactive bladder (OAB) syndrome presents most commonly as urinary urgency, and can be accompanied by frequency and nocturia, with or without urge incontinence, in the absence of urinary tract infection (UTI) or other obvious pathology.

Anal Incontinence

Includes the involuntary passage of gas, mucus, liquid, or solid stool. The most common type of incontinence is watery/liquid stool (>20%), followed by hard and normal stool (approximately 9% for both). The prevalence as suggested by international population-based studies of faecal incontinence is between 0.4 and 18%.

Paradoxical Puborectalis Contraction

The puborectalis muscle, part of the levator ani muscle, wraps like a sling around the lower rectum, acts to control the anorectal angle and consequently facilitates evacuation of bowel content. During a bowel movement, the puborectalis muscle relaxes to allow the bowel contents to pass. If the muscle does not relax and/or contracts paradoxically, it can lead to straining and functional constipation, which is challenging to treat.

Levator Syndrome

Levator syndrome refers to abnormal muscle spasms of the pelvic floor. Spasms may occur after a bowel movement or may be idiopathic. Patients often have long periods of vague, dull, or achy pressure high in the rectum. These symptoms may worsen when sitting or lying down. Levator spasm is more common in women than men.

Coccygodynia

Coccygodynia is pain of the coccyx, usually worsened with movement and after defecation. It is usually caused by trauma to the coccyx, although in a third of patients no cause may be found.

Proctalgia Fugax

This functional disorder is caused by spasms of the rectum and/or the muscles of the pelvic floor, leading to sudden abnormal anal pain that often awakens patients from sleep. This pain may last from a few seconds to several minutes and goes away between episodes.

Pudendal Neuralgia

The pudendal nerves are mixed nerves, with predominant sensory supply to the pelvic floor, external genitalia and perineum. Pudendal neuralgia is chronic pelvic floor pain involving the pudendal nerves. This pain may first occur after childbirth, but often waxes and wanes without reason.

Epidemiology

The prevalence of PFD increases steadily with age. With improved life expectancy, the prevalence and burden of the disorder is bound to increase. The burden of the disease is perceived not just at an individual level but healthcare providers also are affected and the impact on healthcare is likely to increase.

Pelvic Organ Prolapse

About 316 million women suffer from genital prolapse worldwide. Based solely on patient symptoms, the prevalence of pelvic organ prolapse (POP) is 3–6%; however, it rises up to 50% if based on clinical examination because most of the mild cases are asymptomatic. According to the Women's Health Initiative (WHI) in the United States, 40% of women have some degree of POP with 14% having uterine prolapse. The incidence of POP surgery varies from 1.5–1.8 per 1000-woman years with peak age at 60–69. The probability of having a surgical correction for POP by age 80 is estimated to be one in five.

Based on the WHI data, incidence of stage 1–3 prolapse is estimated to be 9.3 per 100 woman-years for cystocele, 5.7 per 100 woman-years for rectocele, and 1.5 per100 woman-years for uterine prolapse. Prolapse progression ranged from 1.9% for uterine prolapse, to 9.5% for cystocele, and 14% for rectocele. Older, parous women are more likely to develop new or progressive prolapse.

In the United States, POP is thought to be the leading cause of more than 300 000 surgical procedures per year with 25% undergoing reoperations at a total cost of more than one billion dollars annually. The estimated direct annual cost of ambulatory care utilisation for pelvic floor disorders during a nine-year period (1996–2005) increased by 40% and, if extrapolated to POP surgery, the total annual cost would be over 1.4 billion.

Urinary Incontinence

UI is more common in women than men and studies from numerous countries have reported the prevalence of UI in women to range from approximately 5–70%, with most studies reporting a prevalence of any UI in the range of 25–45%. In nonpregnant women aged 20 years and above, the prevalence has been reported at 10–17%. These figures increase with increasing age, and in women 65 years and older, more than 50% of the population is affected. The estimated cost of UUI with OAB in the United States during 2007 was $65.9 billion, with projected costs of $76.2 billion in 2015 and $82.6 billion in 2020. With the addition of SUI, this figure may be higher.

Anal Incontinence

The prevalence and epidemiology of anal incontinence is poorly documented and under-reported by patients primarily due to embarrassment and concerns regarding treatment options. The prevalence of faecal incontinence in American women is estimated to impact 2.2–24% depending on the definition used. Severe faecal incontinence, defined as incontinence greater than or equal to one episode monthly, is reported to be present in 6.3% of women.

Furthermore, obstetric anal sphincter injuries in vaginal births are serious complications that share a well-known association with anal incontinence. Injury to the anal sphincter during childbirth approximately doubles the risk of developing anal incontinence within six months after a first delivery.

Predisposing Factors

- **Genetic predisposition**: Women with prolapse were more likely to have positive family history and an increased prevalence of congenital weakness of connective tissue. A systematic review of genetic studies found that collagen type 3 alpha 1 was associated with POP (OR 4.79).
- **Age**: According to The National Institute of Health study, the prevalence of PFD varies from 10% at ages 20–39 years, 27% at 40–59 years, 37% at 60–79 years to nearly 50% affected at 80 years of age and older. The US National Health and Nutrition Examination Survey 2005–2010 stated that the prevalence of faecal incontinence increased from 2.91% among the 20–29 years old to 16.16% among participants 70 years and older.
- **Race**: Although the evidence is scarce, Latin and Caucasian women were found to have a higher risk of symptomatic POP as compared to African American women. Similarly, the age-adjusted prevalence of weekly UI varied based on

ethnicity. Hispanic women had the highest rates, followed by white, black, and Asian American women (36, 30, 25, and 19% respectively, $p > 0.001$). It may be important to note the bias due to the impact of culture-based differences in perception of symptoms.

- **Obesity**: Increased body mass index (BMI) is an independent risk factor for pelvic floor disorders and progression of POP. Weight loss has not been associated with prolapse resolution, but studies have shown that weight loss through lifestyle changes and/or bariatric surgery in overweight or obese women improves both urinary and faecal incontinence.

- **Parity**: Though vaginal birth has been considered the most important inciting factor for pelvic floor disorders, pregnancy itself has been shown to be a risk factor. Studies have shown a direct correlation between the incidence of pelvic floor disorders and parity: 12.8, 18.4, 24.6, and 32.4 for 0, 1, 2, and 3 or more deliveries, respectively ($P < 0.001$). Operative vaginal deliveries and perineal lacerations increase the risk further. Spontaneous vaginal birth as compared to caesarean birth without labour has been associated with higher rates of prolapse or stress incontinence.

- **Smoking**: The Pelvic Organ Support Study (POSST) 2005, revealed that smoking was an independent risk factor for pelvic disorders including POP and UI. The prevalence of prolapse increased significantly amongst nulliparous smokers as compared to nulliparous non-smokers (28vs 12%, adjusted OR 1.95).

- **Medical disorders**: Studies have shown an association between pelvic floor disorders and various medical conditions including diabetes mellitus, connective tissue disorders, chronic obstructive pulmonary disease (COPD), and certain neurological diseases.

- **Coexisting pelvic floor disorders**: Pelvic floor disorders often coexist. Patients with POP often complain of SUI due to obvious reasons. It is often difficult to find patients with any one form of incontinence as most patients have concurrent stress and urge incontinence. Therefore, it is important to analyse these patients thoroughly before formulating a treatment plan.

- **Others**: Traumatic injury to the pelvic region including injuries due to pelvic surgery or pelvic irradiation and heavy lifting are associated with PFD.

Pelvic Organ Support

Pelvic Floor

The pelvic floor consists of muscular and fascial structures. It encloses the pelvic cavity, the external vaginal opening (for intercourse and parturition), and the urethra and rectum (for elimination). The pelvic muscles provide the primary support and with the connective tissue (endopelvic fascia) keep pelvic organs in proper alignment. Together they stabilise, support, and also help in appropriate functioning of the pelvic organs. A sound understanding of the clinical relevance of the bony, muscular, and fascial supports is vital to optimise the surgical techniques in pelvic surgery.

Muscular Support

The levator ani muscle and associated connective tissue attachments constitutes the pelvic diaphragm. It has two main components that function as a unit: the diaphragmatic part (iliococcygeus and coccygeus muscles) and the pubovisceral part (puborectalis and pubococcygeus). The pelvic diaphragm is stretched like a hammock from pubis to coccyx and is attached along the lateral pelvic walls to a thickened band in the obturator fascia, the arcus tendineus levator ani (ATLA).

The iliococcygeus spans from the ATLA between pubis and ischial spine (IS) to insert in the midline onto the anococcygeal raphe and the coccyx. The anococcygeal raphe between the anus and coccyx is referred to as the levator plate and provides support to the uterus, upper vagina, and rectum. The coccygeus muscle originates from the IS and inserts on the lateral lower sacrum and coccyx and overlies the sacrospinous ligament. It often blends with the sacrospinous ligament making it difficult to distinguish the two as they both share a common origin and insertion.

The puborectalis arises from the posterior inferior pubic rami and passes posteriorly forming a U-shaped sling around the vagina, rectum, and perineal body to form the anorectal angle. Some of the fibres of the muscle intermingle with the anal sphincter muscle and contribute to faecal continence. The pubococcygeus has a similar origin, but it inserts in the midline onto the anococcygeal raphe and the anterolateral borders of the coccyx. The openings between the levatorani muscles through which the urethra, vagina, and rectum pass are known as the urogenital hiatus (Figure 2.1).

The pelvic floor muscle fibres maintain resting tone (type I or slow-twitch fibres) to support the pelvic viscera, and voluntarily contract (type II or fast-twitch fibres) when required. It is the skeletal component that contracts to help maintain continence in acute stress states such as cough, laugh, or sneeze. Contraction of the levator ani can be assessed and felt as a U-shaped sling on rectovaginal examination.

The levator ani muscle may get thinner and attenuated with ageing and POP. Neuromuscular injury to the levator, as occurs during childbirth, can lead to widening of the urogenital hiatus, which leads to vertical inclination of the levator plate with resulting pelvic organ dysfunction or POP. Levator avulsion, a documented injury of childbirth, involves the detachment of the puborectalis portion from the pelvic sidewalls. It occurs in about 36% of women after vaginal delivery

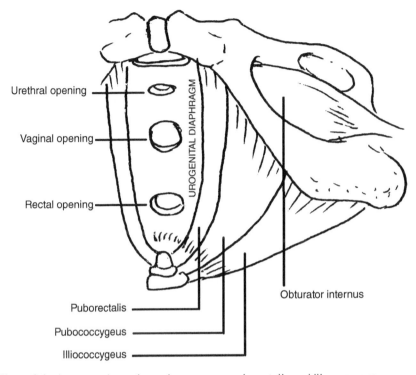

Figure 2.1   Levator ani muscle – pubococcygeus, puborectalis, and iliococcygeus.

and about 50–60% after forceps delivery. Avulsion can be diagnosed digitally by palpating the inferior pubic ramus and feeling for the insertion of the puborectalis portion. In the presence of levator avulsion, 2–3 cm lateral to the urethra, the bony surface of the pubic ramus can be palpated devoid of the muscle.

The perineal body is an important structure that supports the distal vagina and maintains normal rectal function. Lying between the distal vagina and anus, it provides insertion of bulbospongiosus, superficial, and deep transverse perineal muscles, external anal sphincter, perineal membrane, distal part of rectovaginal fascia (RVF), pubococcygeus and puborectalis portions of the levator ani. Surgical reconstruction of perineum (perineorrhaphy) requires proper approximation of these muscles in order to restore the normal function of perineal body (Figure 2.2).

The perineal membrane (formerly known as the urogenital diaphragm) is a thick fibromuscular sheet that stretches across the anterior urogenital triangle. It attaches laterally to the ischiopubic rami and has a free posterior margin with anchorage at the perineal body. The urethra and vagina pass through the hiatus in the perineal membrane. The perineal membrane therefore fixes the distal urethra, distal vagina, and the perineal body to the bony pelvis at the ischiopubic rami. The

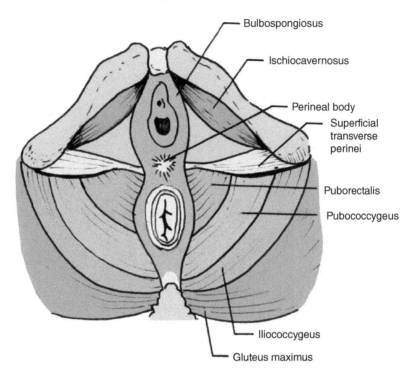

Figure 2.2 Perineal body with its muscular attachments.

superficial perineal space lies external to the perineal membrane and contains the superficial perineal muscles, ischiocavernosus muscle, bulbospongiosus muscle, and superficial transverse perineal muscles.

The deep perineal pouch lies between the perineal membrane and levator ani and contains the external urethral sphincter, the compressor urethra, urethrovaginalis, and the deep transverse perineal muscles (Figure 2.3).

Fascial Support

The parietal and visceral (endopelvic) fascia constitute the fascial components. Parietal fascia covers the pelvic skeletal muscles and provides attachment of muscles to the bony pelvis extending from the lateral pelvic wall to the superior surface of pelvic diaphragm, and it is characterised histologically by regular arrangements of collagen. The obturator fascia covering the obturator muscle has two parts: ATLA and arcus tendineus fascia pelvis (ATFP), extending from IS to posterior pubis. Visceral endopelvic fascia is less discrete and not a true fascia but

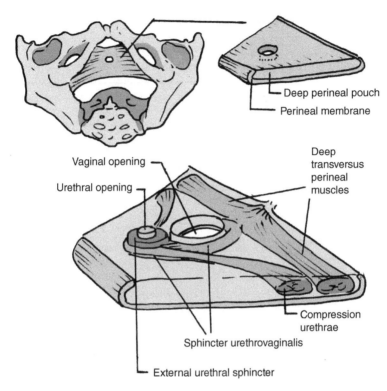

Deep perineal pouch
Perineal membrane

Vaginal opening
Urethral opening

Deep transversus perineal muscles

Compression urethrae

Sphincter urethrovaginalis

External urethral sphincter

Figure 2.3 Muscles of the deep perineal pouch.

is endopelvic connective tissue. It contains a meshwork of loosely arranged collagen, elastin, and adipose tissue through which the blood vessels, lymphatics, and nerves travel to reach the pelvic organs. By surgical convention, condensations of this fascia have been described as discrete 'ligaments', such as the cardinal, uterosacral, pubovisceral, and pubourethral ligaments. The endopelvic tissue is a continuous layer extending from the uterosacral ligaments proximally to the pelvic portion of levator ani muscle distally, up to the level of urethra. The fascia also extends from the lateral wall of the cervix and vagina to the pelvic sidewall along the ATFP. This attachment stretches the vagina horizontally between the bladder and rectum thereby dividing the pelvis into an anterior and posterior compartment. The bladder and urethra occupy the anterior compartment; the rectum and anal canal, the posterior compartment; and the uterus and cervix, the middle or apical compartment.

DeLancey (1994) described the three integrated levels of pelvic support defined by the endopelvic connective tissue attachments to explain POP (see Table 2.1). All are connected through a continuation of the endopelvic fascia (Figure 2.4).

Table 2.1 Level of supports, with diagnosis and co-relation to symptoms.

Level of pelvic organ support	Organ affected	Type of Prolapse	Symptoms
Level I – uterosacral ligaments/ Cardinal ligaments	Uterus and cervix/ vaginal vault	Uterocervical/ vault prolapse/ enterocele	Vaginal pressure, sacral backache, 'something coming down', dyspareunia, vaginal discharge
Level II – arcus tendineus fascia pelvis (ATFP)	Anterior - Urinary bladder	Cystocele	'Something coming down', double voiding, occult stress incontinence, recurrent urinary tract infections
	Posterior – Rectum	Rectocele	'Something coming down', difficult defecation, manual digitation
Level III – anterior (pubourethral ligaments)	Urethra	Urethrocele	'Something coming down', stress incontinence
Level III – posterior (perineal body)	Lower third of the vagina/ vaginal introitus/anal canal	Enlarged genital hiatus	Vaginal laxity, sexual dysfunction, vaginal flatus, needing to apply pressure to the perineum to evacuate faeces

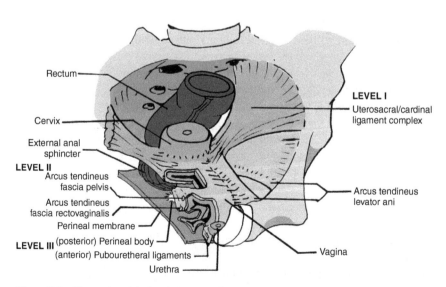

Figure 2.4 The endopelvic fascia in a post-hysterectomy patient divided into DeLancey's biomechanical levels: level I, proximal suspension; level II, lateral attachment; level III, distal fusion.

Level I Support

The cervix and upper vagina are suspended by the endopelvic fascia (parametria) and condensations of the connective tissue, the uterosacral and cardinal ligaments. The uterosacral ligaments pass from the posterior aspect of the cervix and upper vagina, form the lateral boundaries of the pouch of Douglas, and attach to the anterior surface of the sacrum at the level of the sacrococcygeal joint up to the level of S3. The uterosacral ligaments are each 12–14 cm long and subdivided into distal (2–3 cm), intermediate (5 cm), and proximal (5–6 cm). The distal portion is commonly used to anchor the vaginal apex in McCall's culdoplasty. The proximal portion is diffuse in attachment and generally thinner. The intermediate portion is thick, well defined, and at least 2.5 cm away from the ureter and hence suitable for suspension procedures. The cardinal ligaments (transverse cervical) attach to the posterolateral pelvic walls from the cervix and lateral vaginal fornix. These attachments are referred to as the level I or suspensory support. Together, they support the lower uterus, cervix, and upper vagina. They also maintain vaginal length and a nearly horizontal vaginal axis supported by the levator plate. Failure of the level I support leads to uterine or vaginal vault prolapse (apical prolapse).

Level II Support

The fascial attachment in the mid-vagina extends from the lateral vaginal walls to the ATFP anteriorly and arcus tendineus rectovaginalis posteriorly. It maintains the midline position of the vagina directly over the rectum and prevents the descent of the anterior and posterior vaginal walls with increased intra-abdominal pressure. The ATFP shares the same origin as ATLA at the ischial spine. However, it traverses infero-medially to the ATLA before it inserts on the inferior aspect of the superior pubic rami over the origin of the puborectalis muscle. This explains the normal axis of the upper vagina, as the axis of both ATLA and ATFP are nearly horizontal in a standing woman (Figure 2.5). The endopelvic fascia blends with the vaginal muscularis anteriorly, the rectal muscularis posteriorly, and the perineal body inferiorly. The arcus tendineus rectovaginalis is approximately 4 cm in length and changes the axis of the distal vagina towards the vertical.

The endopelvic connective tissue also extends as pubourethral ligaments, from the urethra to the posterior surface of the pubic bone, providing urethral support and maintenance of bladder neck closure during Valsalva manoeuvres. The bladder neck through its relation to the anterior vaginal wall is also indirectly supported by its attachment axis. Hence, failure of level II support leads not only to anterior and posterior vaginal wall prolapse but may also lead to SUI.

The differentiation between a 'central cystocele' and a 'paravaginal defect' in anterior compartment prolapse is based on the type of endopelvic fascia deficiency. In central cystocele (distension cystocele), there is weakening of the

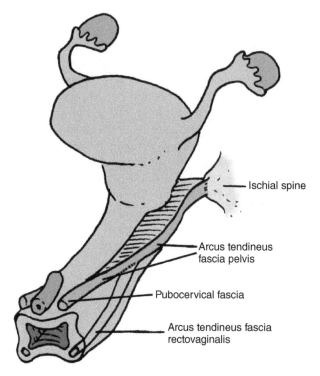

Ischial spine

Arcus tendineus
fascia pelvis

Pubocervical fascia

Arcus tendineus fascia
rectovaginalis

Figure 2.5 The lateral attachments of the pubocervical fascia (PCF) and the rectovaginal fascia (RVF) to the pelvic sidewall. Also shown are the arcus tendineus fascia pelvis (ATFP), arcus tendineus fascia rectovaginalis (ATFRV) and ischial spine (IS).

connective tissue in the midline, resulting in the loss of midline rugosity of the vaginal wall. A lateral cystocele or paravaginal defect results from lateral detachment of the fascia from the ATFP, and the central rugosity is preserved in these. Prior to surgical intervention, it is important to identify the type of anterior wall prolapse as either a lateral detachment or central defect in order to plan the optimal surgical technique.

Level III Support

The lower one-third of the vagina is fused with the surrounding structures through the endopelvic fascia anteriorly to the distal urethra, posteriorly to the perineal body, and laterally to the pubovaginalis muscle and perineal membrane. Together they support and maintain the normal position of the distal one-third of the vagina and introitus. The perineal body is critical for support of the lower part of the vagina and proper function of the anal canal.

Perineal descent can occur due to separation of the anchored perineal membrane from the perineal body and can contribute to defecatory dysfunction. Therefore, level III disruption anteriorly can result in SUI from urethral hypermobility, and posterior disruption can result in distal rectocele or perineal descent.

The endopelvic fascia becomes the primary mechanism of support in circumstances when neuropathic injury or mechanical damage leads to pelvic floor muscle weakness. This may lead to loss of normal anatomic position if the ongoing stress overcomes the strength of the endopelvic fascial attachments. The resultant altered vector forces may lead to POP and/or visceral dysfunction. The goal of reconstructive pelvic surgery should be to recreate these supportive connections and restore the anatomical position of the pelvic organs while maintaining adequate vaginal length to maintain the vaginal apex in a natural position.

Conclusion

A thorough understanding of pelvic anatomy is necessary prior to planning any urogynaecological procedure. The types of pelvic floor disorders and being aware of the risk factors help the surgeon in planning the appropriate surgery.

Further Reading

Abrams, P., Cardozo, L., Fall, M. et al. (2002). The standardisation of terminology of lower urinary tract function: report from the Standardisation Subcommittee of the International Continence Society. *Neurourol and Urodyn.* 21 (2): 167–178.

DeLancey, J.O. (1994 Aug). The anatomy of the pelvic floor. *Current Opinion in Obstetrics & Gynecology* 6 (4): 313–316.

DeLancey, J.O.L. (2003). Functional anatomy of the pelvic floor. In: *Imaging Pelvic Floor Disorders* (eds. C.I. Bartram and J.O.L. DeLancey), 27–38. Berlin, Heidelberg: Springer.

Iglesia, C.B. and Smithling, K.R. (2017). Pelvic organ prolapse. *Am. Fam. Physician* 96 (3): 179–185.

MichiganUo (2018). Urinary Incontinence: an inevitable part of aging? National Poll on Health Aging. http://www.healthyagingpoll.org/sites/default/files/2018-11/ NPHA_Incontinence-Report_

Whitcomb, E.L., Rortveit, G., Brown, J.S. et al. (2009). Racial differences in pelvic organ prolapse. *Obstet. Gynecol.* 114 (6): 1271–1277.

3

Ambulatory Evaluation of Pelvic Organ Prolapse and Urinary Incontinence

Tanvir Singh, Sandhya Gupta, and Ajay Rane

This chapter deals with the role of different ambulatory practices in the evaluation of pelvic organ prolapse (POP) and urinary incontinence (UI). A good history combined with a proper clinical examination is simple, inexpensive, and a time saving tool, in the diagnosis of pelvic floor disorders. This leaves very few women requiring sophisticated tests for evaluation and management.

History

Presenting Symptoms

The aim of eliciting a complete description of the nature of the patient's symptoms is to put together a working diagnosis and gauge the impact of the symptoms on the patient's quality of life. While taking a history, it is important to define the most troublesome symptom and the patient's expectations from the treatment.

Urinary Incontinence (UI) is the complaint of any involuntary leakage of urine. It is a storage symptom and should be described by specifying relevant factors such as type, onset, frequency, severity, progression/regression, precipitating factors, social impact, effect on hygiene and quality of life, response or non-response to treatment, the measures used to contain the leakage (wearing of protection) and whether the individual seeks or desires help because of UI. Urinary leakage may need to be distinguished from other causes of wetness such as sweating or vaginal discharge.

Ambulatory Urology and Urogynaecology, First Edition. Edited by Abhay Rane and Ajay Rane.

Stress Urinary Incontinence (SUI) is the complaint of involuntary leakage on effort or exertion—for example, lifting heavy weights, jumping, or on sneezing or coughing.

Urge Urinary Incontinence (UUI) is the complaint of involuntary leakage accompanied by or immediately preceded by urgency. Information on triggering events such as cold, running water and 'latch key' incontinence should be noted.

Mixed Urinary Incontinence (MUI) is the complaint of involuntary leakage associated with urgency and also with exertion, sneezing, or coughing.

Nocturnal Enuresis is the complaint of loss of urine occurring during sleep. History of previous childhood nocturnal enuresis and delayed bladder control in childhood is associated with detrusor overactivity (DO) or overflow incontinence in adulthood.

Continuous Urinary Incontinence is the complaint of continuous urinary leakage, usually suggestive of urinary fistula.

Urological History

There is usually an overlap of symptoms with stress, urge, and mixed incontinence. A careful history should be obtained regarding frequency, urgency, dysuria, and nocturia. UI symptoms of recent onset, combined with irritative bladder symptoms, should prompt investigation for an infective cause. To evaluate a patient with incontinence, objective tools to use include the incontinence specific quality-of-life scales or validated questionnaires. These allow evaluation of the severity and the relative contribution of UUI and SUI symptoms and the response to their therapies. The following questionnaires have good test–retest reliability: The International Consultation on Incontinence Questionnaire (ICIQ), Bristol Female Lower Urinary Tract Symptoms (BFLUTS), Incontinence Quality Of Life (I-QOL), Stress and Urge Incontinence Quality of life Questionnaire (SUIQQ), Urinary Incontinence Severity Score (UISS), The Stress related leak, Emptying ability, Anatomy, Protection, Inhibition, Quality of life, Mobility and Mental status (SEAPI-QMM), and The King's Health Questionnaire (KHQ).

Pelvic Organ Prolapse (POP)

The preferred system to describe and document the POP is the Pelvic Organ Prolapse Quantification (POPQ) system. Over the years, many clinicians have familiarised themselves with the POPQ and use it in their daily practice. The symptomatology of POP, apart from pelvic mass, can be related to bladder or bowel disturbance symptoms. The presenting feature can therefore be a combination of any of the following symptoms, and it is important to elicit the history accordingly.

Bulge Symptoms

Bulge/mass at the vaginal introitus
Pelvic or vaginal pressure
Bearing down sensation
Feeling of something falling out

Urinary Symptoms

UI/frequency/urgency
Dysuria
Pain on bladder filling
Weak or prolonged urinary stream
Hesitancy

Bowel Symptoms

Rectal tenesmus or constipation
Digital splinting to defecate

Pain

Lower back discomfort or vulval discomfort
Pain in the vagina, bladder, or rectum

Sexual Symptoms

Difficult intercourse due to the mass
Vaginal looseness
Dyspareunia
Decreased lubrication/Vaginal dryness
Decreased arousal or orgasm
Vaginal flatus

Bowel Habits

Bowel dysfunction frequently affects urinary function. Constipation is the second most important predisposing factor for UI after vaginal birth. UI may coexist with faecal incontinence, and most women are hesitant to talk about this symptom. One study evaluated 247 women with either UI or POP and found that 31% of women with UI and 7% with POP had concurrent anal incontinences. For these reasons, women should be specifically asked about anal incontinence including the type of loss, such as flatus, liquid stool or solid stool and the frequency.

General Medical History

The initial history includes a review of medical problems, current medications, and history of pelvic surgeries. Medical conditions can influence bladder function and symptoms. Some drugs can worsen incontinence (Table 3.1). Neurological conditions such as multiple sclerosis may cause overflow incontinence and urinary retention. Visual impairment and immobility such as severe arthritis makes it difficult for the patient to reach the toilet in time. In addition, obesity, smoking, constipation, and work involving heavy lifting can chronically increase intra-abdominal

Table 3.1 Effects of common medications on bladder functions.

Medication	Mechanism	Bladder dysfunction
Cough and cold preparations Pseudoephedrine, ephedrine, phenylpropanolamine	Increase urethral closure pressure	Urinary retention
Antihypertensive agents Prazosin, terazosin, methyldopa, reserpine, guanethidine	Alpha adrenergic antagonists decrease urethral pressure	Worsen stress urinary incontinence
Diuretics Thiazides, loop diuretics, alcohol	Increase urinary output	Worsen urinary frequency/urge incontinence
Anticholinergic agents Antihistamines, tricyclic antidepressants	Detrusor relaxation	Urinary retention
Antiparkinson agents Benztropine, trihexyphenidyl	Detrusor relaxation	Urinary retention
Beta-blockers Pindolol, disospyramide	Detrusor relaxation	Urinary retention
Antipsychotic agents Haloperidol, thioridazine	Alpha adrenergic antagonists decrease urethral pressure	Urinary retention
Calcium channel blockers Verapamil	Detrusor relaxation	Urinary retention
Iron, narcotics, sedatives	Constipation	
ACE inhibitors Enalapril	Indirect cough effects	

pressure, which can worsen urinary symptoms. Obesity in women is associates with a threefold increased risk of UI compared to non-obese women. Caffeine intake, diabetes, stroke, depression, faecal incontinence, genitourinary syndrome of menopause, vaginal atrophy, hormone replacement therapy, radiation, pelvic surgeries including hysterectomy are some of the other risk factors.

It is important to consider conditions outside the urinary tract that may influence continence. Treating these conditions often restores continence. Functional causes of incontinence as been summarised using the acronym 'DIAPPERS' (Resnick):

D = Delirium
I = Infection
A = Atrophic urethritis or vaginitis
P = Pharmacologic agents
P = Psychiatric disorders
E = Excess urinary output (e.g. congestive heart failure, hyperglycaemia)
R = Restricted mobility or dexterity
S = Stool impaction

Obstetric History

UI in pregnancy is reported by 7–60% of women and in most, will resolve after delivery. Parity, mode of delivery including instrumental deliveries, and birth weight, are some identifiable risk factors in both UI and POP.

Vaginal delivery is identified as an independent risk factor for prolapse. This risk increases with forceps delivery, with increasing parity and in women having their first child at a later age. Caesarean delivery however does not appear to be protective.

Gynaecological History

Presence of a pelvic mass, such as fibroids or ovarian cysts, and the menopausal status is also relevant. In several studies, the prevalence of pelvic floor disorders has been shown to increase with menopause. The prevalence of any one pelvic floor disorder with menopause was estimated to be 37%, which included SUI 15%, OAB 13%, POP 6% and anal incontinence 25%.

Family History

The existence of inherited risk factors for pelvic floor disorders has long been recognised and there is a clear familial aggregation for these conditions. Having an affected first-degree relative with incontinence or prolapse is associated with an approximately two- to threefold increased risk of developing either condition. A study looking at twins, attributed a 35–55% genetic contribution to urge incontinence/overactive bladder but only 1.5% for stress incontinence.

Quality of Life

A more objective tool to assess the quality of life would be to use the incontinence specific scales or validated patient questionnaires. The Modified Bristol Female Lower Urinary Tract Symptoms Questionnaire can be used to evaluate the severity of UUI and SUI symptoms and the response to their therapies. The Pelvic Floor Distress Inventory (PFDI) and the Pelvic Floor Impact Questionnaire (PFIQ) can assess the urinary, colorectal, and prolapse symptoms in detail. The International Consultation on Incontinence Questionnaire and the Kings Health questionnaire are available for evaluating impact of incontinence on quality of life. The Patient Global Impression of Improvement (PGII) and Patient Global Impression of Severity (PGIS) are also acceptable measures to assess improvement and satisfaction, respectively.

Sexual Dysfunction

Coital incontinence may occur during arousal, on penetration, throughout intercourse, or specifically on orgasm. Urodynamic stress incontinence (USI) is the most common urodynamic finding; however, DO is found more often when leakage is restricted to orgasm. It is therefore helpful to define when urine leakage occurs during these acts. Up to 68% of women report that their sex life is ruined due to urinary symptoms.

Physical Examination

General Examination

A general physical examination includes assessment of a women's body mass index (BMI), identification of mobility restriction or visual impairment, and the odour of urine, smoke, or alcohol. The information gained from these observations needs to be addressed and modified for the success of any treatment.

Neurological Examination

All patients should have a neurological evaluation and it begins with the assessment of mental status. Bladder dysfunction is common in patients with dementia, stroke, parkinsonism, multiple sclerosis, and hence, facial symmetry, gait, dexterity and speech pattern should be noted. In cognitively impaired patients, a family member or friend should be present during examination to improve the compliance.

The neurological control of bladder storage and voiding function necessitates assessment of the thoraco-lumbar and sacral segments of the spinal cord. Motor strength, deep tendon reflexes, lower limb sensation and the sacral reflexes – bulbo cavernous and anal reflex – can identify neurological problems.

Abdominal Examination

This examination is particularly important to identify abdominal masses such as fibroids or ovarian cysts, which can compress on the bladder causing frequency, urgency, UI, or obstruction. Suprapubic tenderness may indicate infective aetiology or a urinary tract stone. Along with the evaluation of masses, scars, and organomegaly, the integrity of the abdominal wall should be assessed. Abdominal wall defects such as diastasis recti can influence the symptoms of stress incontinence and prolapse.

External Gynaecological Examination

Inspection of the vulva and perineum is often the neglected part of the gynaecological examination. It is important to look for excoriation and erythema due to incontinence and the use of pads. Clinician should also look for signs of hypoestrogenism (Figure 3.1) such as atrophy of the vulvar skin, agglutination of the labia minora (Figure 3.2) or urethral caruncle.

The clinical sign of UI is defined as urine leakage seen during examination, which may be urethral or extra-urethral. Extra-urethral incontinence is defined as urine leakage from a site other than urethra, such as ectopic ureter (congenital) or urogenital fistula.

External examination also involves identifying level III support defects such as measurement of the genital hiatus (normal 4–6 cm in length) and of the perineal body (normal 2–4 cm in length). In POP, assessment of level I and level II defects is required and is further described in the following section.

The perineal body is attached anteriorly to the perineal membrane and cranially to the posterior vaginal wall. This cranial attachment causes the perineum to be concave and limits its downward mobility to about 1 cm. Perineal descent is characterised by bulging and widening of the perineum during Valsalva, with the perineal body movement being greater than 2 cm below the level of ischial tuberosities. On POPQ examination this is identified by widening of genital hiatus and shortening of perineal body. With complete disruption of the perineal muscles, a perineal rectocele develops. When this occurs, the perineal body elongates and demonstrates ballooning on Valsalva.

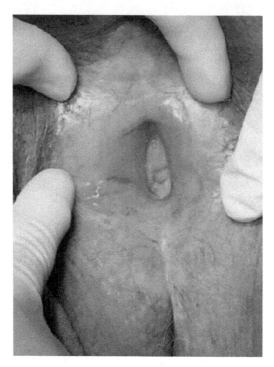

Figure 3.1 Signs of hypoestrogenism, scarcity of pubic hair, loss of elasticity of skin, dryness of labia, introital stenosis, vulvar erythema. *Source:* With permission from Dr Meeta and patient.

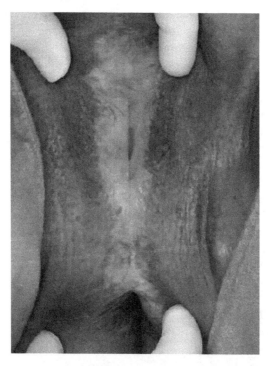

Figure 3.2 Labial fusion due to genito urinary syndrome of menopause (GSM). *Source:* With permission from Dr Meeta and patient.

Internal Gynaecological Examination

A speculum examination of the vagina is needed to evaluate for atrophy and POP. The woman is examined at rest and at maximum Valsalva, while in the supine position with the legs comfortably flexed. DeLancey has defined three levels of support of pelvic organs – Level I, Level II, and Level III, which is accepted worldwide. On speculum examination, prolapse of each level and each compartment is evaluated as follows:

- Apical prolapse or Level I (prolapse of the cervix or vaginal vault) – A bivalve speculum is inserted into the vagina and then slowly withdrawn, any descent of the apex (cervix, vault) is noted.
- Anterior vaginal wall or Level II – A Sims retractor or the posterior blade of a bivalve speculum is inserted into the vagina with gentle pressure on the posterior vaginal wall to isolate and visualise the anterior vaginal wall.
- Posterior vaginal wall or Level II – A Sims retractor or the posterior blade of a bivalve speculum inserted into the vagina with gentle pressure on the anterior vaginal wall to isolate and visualise the posterior vaginal wall.
- Perineum or Level III – Evaluation involves measurement of the genital hiatus and perineal body and identification of stress urinary incontinence.

Staging of the extent of prolapse is done using a Simplified POPQ validated against original staging system of POPQ:

Stage 1: Prolapse where the given point remains at least 1 cm above the hymenal remnants (see Figure 3.3).

Stage 2: Prolapse where the given point descends to the introitus, defined as an area extending from 1 cm above to 1 cm below the hymenal remnants (see Figure 3.4).

Stage 3: Prolapse where the given point descends greater than 1 cm past the hymenal remnants, but does not represent complete vaginal vault eversion or complete uterine procidentia. This implies that at least some portion of the vaginal mucosa is not everted (Figure 3.5).

Stage 4: Complete vaginal vault eversion or complete uterine procidentia. This implies that the vagina and/or uterus are maximally prolapsed with essentially the entire extent of the vaginal mucosa everted.

At the end of the speculum assessment, bimanual examination is performed to evaluate the uterus and adnexa for enlargement and any masses. Finally, a rectal examination to evaluate the tone and integrity of the anal sphincter may be needed.

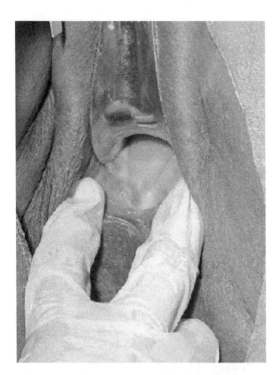

Figure 3.3 Evaluation of posterior vaginal wall prolapse in Valsalva demonstrating Stage 1 Posterior wall POP.

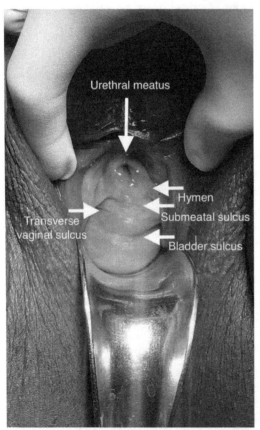

Urethral meatus

Hymen

Submeatal sulcus

Transverse vaginal sulcus

Bladder sulcus

Figure 3.4 Evaluation of anterior vaginal wall prolapse in Valsalva demonstrating Stage 2 Anterior wall POP.

Figure 3.5 Evaluation of anterior vaginal wall prolapse in Valsalva demonstrating Stage 3 Anterior wall POP.

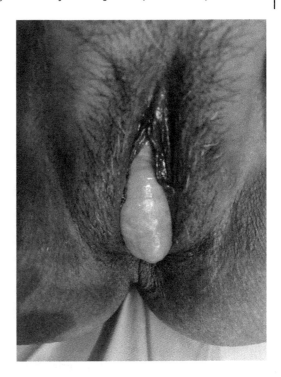

Assessment of Pelvic Muscle Function

Digital assessment of the bony architecture, muscle mass, connective tissue support, pelvic floor muscle contraction and grading using the modified Oxford grading scale (Table 3.2) can be helpful in discussing management options such as pelvic floor exercises.

Table 3.2 Modified Oxford grading scale for pelvic floor muscle strength.

Grade	Definition
0	No contraction
1	Flicker of contraction
2	Weak muscle activity
3	Moderate muscle contraction
4	Good muscle contraction
5	Strong muscle contraction

Investigations

The diagnosis of pelvic floor disorders is often clinical, based on history and examination. This is particularly true in the case of POP. Diagnostic tests and investigations are aimed mainly to assess the severity or rule out co-existing problems.

Urinary Diary

A urinary diary is an inexpensive tool that is easy to keep and interpret. It may suggest a diagnosis and allows conservative treatment to be started. The patient records the type and amount of fluid intake, episodes of incontinence, times voided, and volume of urine voided. Though frequency and volume are neither specific nor sensitive in determining the cause of incontinence, it guides behavioural modification. Ideally a three-day voiding diary to assess outcomes of treatment is suggested in most clinical studies, but compliance is better with a 24-hour diary. Normal voiding frequency is less than eight times a day and once at night, with total volumes of less than 1800 ml per 24 hours.

Urine Analysis

Urinalysis is a fundamental and frequently performed test that determines any evidence of hematuria, pyuria, glycosuria, or proteinuria. Urinary tract infections (UTI) can be identified using urinalysis and treated before initiating further investigations or therapeutic interventions for UI. If the urinalysis tests positive for both leucocytes and nitrites, a midstream urine specimen is sent for microscopy, culture and analysis of antibiotic sensitivity. If symptomatic, these women can be prescribed an appropriate course of antibiotic pending culture results. If women do not have symptoms of a UTI, but their urine tests positive for both leucocytes and nitrites, do not offer antibiotics without the results of midstream urine culture. It is worth noting that 60% of women with a stable bladder will develop DO at the time of a UTI. A urine specimen is sent for cytology if there is haematuria or irritative voiding symptoms to rule out a malignancy. Haematuria consisting of more than 5–10 red cells per high-power field warrants further investigations by imaging and cystoscopy.

Cough Stress Test

A cough stress test (CST) is used in the evaluation of women with SUI. It is an objective test to diagnose and assess the outcome of treatment of SUI syndrome (SUI–S).

The ICS-Uniform Cough Stress Test (ICS-UCST) has standardised the technique of the CST. It recommends that the patient be in a supine/lithotomy position with 200–400 ml of fluid in the bladder. She coughs forcefully one to four times and the examiner directly visualises the urethral meatus for the presence of leakage. Leakage of fluid from the urethral meatus coincident with/ simultaneous to the cough(s) is considered a positive test. Upright CST: If the supine/lithotomy position ICS-UCST is negative, the patient undergoes a repeat test in upright or standing position. It is reported as a positive upright CST.

Supine empty stress test (SEST): A positive CST performed in the supine position with an 'empty' bladder (volume < 100 ml) has been suggested to indicate the presence of intrinsic sphincter deficiency (ISD). In a prospective series it was noted that a positive SEST was associated with a lower maximum urethral closure pressure (MUCP) (mean, 20 vs. 36 cm H_2O). SEST had sensitivity of 65–70% and specificity of 67–76% for predicting ISD. The IUGA suggests that a SEST could be used as a simple test to be reasonably assured that ISD is not present (without resorting to multichannel urodynamics). In a patient with SUI, a negative ICS-UCST can be reassessed with an ICS standard pad test and/or urodynamic testing to completely evaluate the lower urinary tract function, as per current practice guidelines.

Urethro-Vesical Mobility

Support to the bladder neck is assessed by evaluating the mobility of the urethro-vesical junction. Urethral hypermobility is defined as a 30° or greater displacement of the urethra from the horizontal (measured with a cotton tip swab in the urethra). The test, referred to as the 'Q-tip test', is performed in the supine lithotomy position and at maximum Valsalva effort. The angle is measured using a goniometer.

Other methods of evaluating urethral mobility include measurement of point Aa of the POPQ system, visualisation (inaccurate method), ultrasonography, and lateral cystourethrogram. Women with stress incontinence who have demonstrated urethral hypermobility have a lower risk of failure after a mid-urethral sling procedure. In women with SUI without urethral hypermobility, where leak can be due to ISD, bulking agents were considered to be a more appropriate surgical option. This notion is however being increasingly questioned with use of mid-urethral slings, where cure rate of 77% is quoted with tension-free vaginal tape (TVT) in patients with ISD.

Pad Test

The pad test is a non-invasive diagnostic test, which is low cost, simple to perform, and gives both qualitative (presence or absence of UI) and quantitative assessment (determination of degree of UI). The ICS has standardised the pad test both for one-hour and 24-hour testing. In the one-hour pad test, the bladder is filled to a set starting volume of about 150–300 ml of fluid through instillation. A pre-weighed pad is put on by the patient, without voiding. The patient drinks 500 ml of sodium-free liquid in <15 minutes and then sits or rests. Then, the patient walks for 30 minutes, including climbing one flight of stairs (up and down) before performing the following activities: standing up from sitting (10 times), coughing vigorously (10 times), running on the spot for one minute, bending to pick up an object from the floor (five times), and washing their hands in running water for one minute. The total amount of urine leaked is determined by weighing the pad and a weight gain of >1.4 g (equal to 1.4 ml) is significant. If a moderately full bladder cannot be maintained through the hour (if the patient must void), the test has to be started again.

The 24-hour pad test should be started with an empty bladder. The normal daily activities should be followed and recorded in a voiding diary so that the same schedule will be observed during follow-up re-testing. To avoid urine loss through leakage or evaporation, the pads should be worn inside waterproof underpants and changed every four to six hours during daytime. The pads should be weighed immediately, and if weighing is to be performed at the clinic, the pads must be stored in an airtight bag. A weight gain of >4.4 g (equal to 4.4 ml) is considered significant, in a 24-hour test. An increase of 4–20 g/24 hour is classified as representing mild incontinence, 21–74 g/24-hour represents moderate incontinence and >75 g/24-hour represents severe incontinence. The 24-hour pad test, is more reproducible than a one-hour test, but it is highly dependent on patient compliance and therefore not suitable for all patients.

Urogynaecological Ultrasound

The diagnostic utility of ultrasound in imaging pelvic floor disorders is limited to certain specific pathologies but can nonetheless prove to be invaluable. Ultrasound of the abdomen and pelvis, combined with assessment of post-void residual urine volume, can help in ruling out pelvic masses, identifying upper urinary tract dilatation and any voiding problem.

Three- and four-dimensional trans-labial/trans-perineal ultrasonography is a relatively new imaging modality with high accuracy in the evaluation of pelvic floor disorders such as UI, POP, and levator avulsion. A two-dimensional ultrasound can also be used to confirm which compartment a prolapse may be of. Evaluation of mesh implants is another important indication for this modality.

A trans labial ultrasound is used in the assessment of bladder wall thickness, bladder neck and mid-urethral mobility, and funnelling of bladder neck, in women with UI. A two-dimensional mid-sagittal image at rest helps in assessing the post-void residual urine volume.

During Valsalva, the hiatal dimension is measured and a value of less than $25\,mm^2$ at Valsalva is unlikely to be associated with POP. The extent of ballooning, defined as excessive distention of the hiatus, is categorised as mild ($25.0–29.9\,cm^2$), moderate ($30.0–34.9\,cm^2$, marked ($35.0–39.9\,cm^2$), or severe ($\geq40\,cm^2$). POP can be evaluated and quantified with trans-labial scans in all three pelvic compartments.

The endoanal scan performed with a high-resolution probe is considered the reference standard for sphincter evaluation. However, the use of transvaginal probes placed exo-anally in the coronal plane has been accepted for anal sphincter evaluation at rest and during contraction. The normal mucosa is visualised as a hyperechoic area surrounded by a hypoechoic ring that represents the internal anal sphincter. The more external hyperechoic tissue represents the external anal sphincter. Anal sphincter injuries appear as discontinuity of the rings of the internal and external anal sphincter and the clock face is used to report the locations of these injuries (Figure 3.6).

Uroflowmetry

Uroflowmetry is a non-invasive measurement of the rate of urine flow over time. It measures the maximum flow rate, average flow rate, voided volume and gives the flow pattern. It also gives us post-void residual volume, but cannot be used

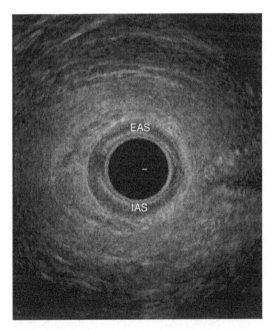

Figure 3.6 Endoanal Scan (IAS – Internal Anal Sphincter, EAS – External Anal Sphincter).

alone to diagnose the cause of an abnormality. The patient is asked to void into a specially designed commode that measures voided volume, maximal, and average urinary flow rates. Uroflowmetry is usually used to determine obstructive voiding. The International Continence Society (ICS) has not defined normal voiding ranges according to maximum flow rate (Qmax) in healthy women (Figure 3.7).

Urodynamic Testing (UDS)

Urodynamics and cystoscopy are not essential in the initial assessment of patients presenting with uncomplicated UI. The role of urodynamics before prolapse surgery is contentious and there is no universal consensus in women with concomitant SUI. UDS could facilitate counselling of patients; however, there is no evidence that the testing alters the outcome of surgery.

The term *urodynamics* encompasses a number of varied physiological tests of bladder and urethral function, which aim to demonstrate an underlying abnormality of storage or voiding. Urodynamics should be used selectively in women with UI to answer specific functional questions. It is important to rule out urinary infection prior to this invasive testing. After undertaking a detailed clinical history and examination, multichannel filling and voiding cystometry are indicated in women who have

- Symptoms suggestive of voiding dysfunction
- OAB symptoms refractory to pharmacotherapy
- Symptoms of OAB with uncertain aetiology or a clinical suspicion of neurogenic DO prior to surgical intervention in women with SUI
- Urinary symptoms following anti-incontinence procedure

Cystometry is a useful method for assessing detrusor muscle function and of bladder symptoms in relation to storage and voiding. Following a uroflowmetry and measurement of the post-void residual urine volume, cystometry is commenced. Cystometry, can be either a single channel cystometry or, more commonly, multichannel cystometry.

In multi-channel cystometry, bladder and rectal/vaginal lines are inserted and residual urine if any, is noted. The bladder is filled at a rate of 50 ml/min and the filling medium is usually normal saline or sterile water at room temperature. The aim is to replicate the woman's symptoms by filling the bladder and observing the pressure changes. The pressure from the bladder is termed Pves or vesical pressure and the Pabd or abdominal pressure is recorded from the rectal/vaginal line. The detrusor pressure Pdet is calculated by subtracting the abdominal from vesical pressure. (Pdet = Pves – Pabd).

Bladder storage functions obtained with filling cystometry include bladder sensation, cystometric bladder capacity, compliance, and presence of involuntary

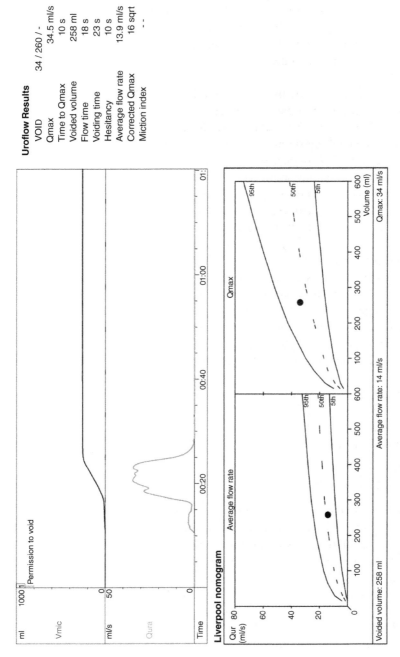

Uroflow Results

VOID	34 / 260 / -
Qmax	34.5 ml/s
Time to Qmax	10 s
Voided volume	258 ml
Flow time	18 s
Voiding time	23 s
Hesitancy	10 s
Average flow rate	13.9 ml/s
Corrected Qmax	16 sqrt
Miction index	- -

Figure 3.7 Uroflowmetry in a healthy woman with stress urinary incontinence. A normal 'bell shaped' curve.

detrusor contractions. Urinary leak demonstrable with cough or Valsalva during filling cystometry is referred to as USI. Presence of involuntary detrusor contractions during filling, associated with urgency and/or leak is referred to as DO. The first desire to void occurs when intravesical pressure is usually about 150 ml and a strong desire at 400 ml in the normal bladder. The average bladder has a capacity of 250–550 ml.

In voiding cystometry, the patient is asked to void once maximum bladder capacity is reached or if patient requests permission to void. Voiding takes place with the lines in situ for pressure recording. The important aspects in voiding cystometry include maximum flow rate, the detrusor pressure, the voided volume, and presence of abdominal straining. An underactive (hypotonic) detrusor is diagnosed when voiding occurs with a slow urine flow rate and low detrusor pressure. In women, obstruction is defined as a peak flow rate of less than 15 ml/s with a maximum voiding detrusor pressure greater than 60 cm of H_2O.

Video-urodynamics involves synchronous radiographic screening of the bladder with multi-channel cystometry using radio-opaque dye as filling medium. Anatomical abnormalities such as diverticulae and reflux can be visualised, and that visualisation is useful in identifying an open bladder neck and proximal urethra. Ambulatory urodynamics involves multi-channel cystometry carried out with physiological bladder filling rates and using portable recording devices, which enable the woman to remain ambulant during the test.

A systematic review of 99 studies including over 80 000 women found insufficient evidence to support the ability of urodynamic testing to predict the outcomes of nonsurgical treatment for stress incontinence. In addition, no improvement in surgical outcomes was demonstrated in a randomised multi-centre trial of preoperative urodynamic testing for uncomplicated stress incontinence. Urodynamics is an invasive test and has to be used judiciously to provide reliable information and to be cost-effective.

Urethral Pressure Profile

There are numerous tests for urethral function, including urethral pressure profilometry and leak point pressure measurement. Intravesical pressure and the intraluminal urethral pressure are measured simultaneously using pressure transducers that are about 5 cm apart. The pressures are measured during filling and during Valsalva. These are used to derive values that reflect the ability of the urethra to resist urine flow, expressed most commonly as maximum urethral closure pressure (MUCP) or as abdominal, cough, or Valsalva leak point pressures (ALPP, CLPP, VLPP, respectively). A MUCP less than 20 cm H_2O denotes ISD and a high MUCP may denote urethral obstruction or diverticulae. ALPP measures the bladder pressure at leak generated by Valsalva and is dynamic in nature. This is used as an indirect measure of the urethral sphincter function. Leakage at an ALPP of less than 60 cm of H_2O is diagnostic of ISD.

Cystoscopy

Cystoscopy is the direct visualisation of the bladder and urethral lumen using either a rigid or flexible cystoscope. A flexible cystoscope is preferable to the rigid for diagnostic purpose, because it can obviate the need for anaesthesia. Cystoscopy may be of value in women with pain or recurrent UTIs, following previous pelvic surgery or where fistula is suspected. Its role in recurrent SUI without these additional features is less clear. Cystoscopic examination is used to identify areas of inflammation (interstitial cystitis), tumours, stones, foreign body, and diverticula, all of which are findings that will require management within a different clinical pathway. Cystoscopy is contraindicated in the presence of an acute cystitis and in patients with severe coagulopathy.

Conclusion

In the evaluation of UI and with the bladder being an 'unreliable witness', several tests have been postulated either to assess the severity or delineate the problem. However, prior to any testing, an appropriate questionnaire, a directed history, and thorough examination must be done. Choosing the appropriate test forms the core of the initial clinical assessment. In POP, diagnosis is mainly clinical, with investigations required only to evaluate any co-existing bladder or bowel problems. In long standing stage IV POP, anatomical and functional assessment of the renal tract with ultrasound imaging and renal function tests may be needed. Anal dysfunction diagnosis, relies on imaging to assess any structural problems in the anal sphincter and anal manometry to assess its function.

Further Reading

Abrams, P., Cardozo, L., Fall, M. et al. (2002). Standardisation of terminology of lower urinary tract function: report from the standardisation sub-committee of the international continence society. *Neurourology and Urodynamics* 21: 167–178.

Avery, K., Donovan, J., Peters, T.J. et al. (2004). ICIQ: a brief and robust measure for evaluating the symptoms and impact of urinary incontinence. *Neurourology and Urodynamics* 23: 322.

Tamilselvi, A. and Rane, A. (eds.) (2015). *Principles and Practice of Urogynaecology*. India: Springer https://doi.org/10.1007/978-81-322-1692-6-5.

Weber, A.M., Abrams, P., Brubaker, L. et al. (2001). The standardization of terminology for researchers in female pelvic floor disorders. *International Urogynecology Journal* 12 (3): 178–186.

4

Role of Cystoscopy

Arjunan Tamilselvi

Cystoscopy is an important armamentarium in the hands of the urologists, urogynaecologists, and gynaecologists. Origins of the cystoscope, follows the endoscopy path, where instruments were designed to peer into the human internal organs. Philip Bozzini, a young obstetrician, is credited with the honour of being the forerunner in designing endoscopy. In 1806, he designed an instrument to be passed through orifices, to inspect the internal organs using candle as light source. Bozzini's Lichtleiter did not break ground with the medical community at that time. This was followed by attempts of several people to rework on the Bozzini design principle to create an endoscope. The next major breakthrough in cystoscopy was achieved by the combined work of a German urologist, Maximilian Nitze, and an instrument maker from Vienna, Joseph Leiter.

The Nitze–Leiter Cystoscope was a success and with the invention of light bulbs in 1880, the cystoscope was well on its way to become part of the surgical practice. Modifications to the Nitze model continued with use of different optics, incorporating catheterization units, operating units, diathermy units, and several others as deemed necessary for the operator. The use of fibre optics revolutionised cystoscopy, providing good visualisation and clear photographs of the bladder.

Cystoscopic examination currently uses either a rigid or flexible cystoscope and is employed either for diagnostic or therapeutic procedures. Cystoscopy is one of the procedures ideally suited to be done in an ambulatory set-up.

Instrument

A rigid cystoscope consists of a metal sheath, obturator, bridge, and telescope to which the light source is attached (Figure 4.1).The sheath has channels for irrigation fluid, and the bridge can have one or two working channels for insertion of

Ambulatory Urology and Urogynaecology, First Edition. Edited by Abhay Rane and Ajay Rane.
© 2021 John Wiley & Sons Ltd. Published 2021 by John Wiley & Sons Ltd.

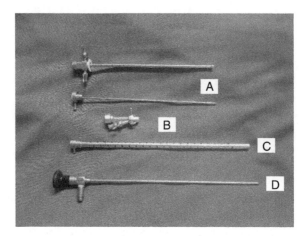

Figure 4.1 Rigid Cystoscope. (A) Sheath with irrigation channels and obturator. (B) Bridge. (C) Sheath cover. (D) Telescope.

instruments. Cystoscope sizes are given in French scale and refer to the outside diameter of the sheath in millimetres. (1 Fr = 0.3 mm, 15 Fr = 5 mm). The diameter of the sheath that is used commonly in adults is 17–24 French. In selected cases, a paediatric cystoscope may be needed (8 French).

Irrigation fluid in a cystoscope is usually sterile water or normal saline. If any electro-coagulation is planned, electrolyte containing solutions must be avoided. Fluid distension in cystoscopy is gravity based with the fluid bag, placed minimum 80 cm above the patient position.

Different types of lenses are used in cystoscope and the operator chooses them according to the area to be visualised. A 0° or 12° lens is usually used for inspection of urethra, but are not particularly useful for visualisation of entire bladder. A 30° lens is useful in the visualisation of the posterior wall and base of the bladder and helpful in ureteric catheterization or stent insertion. A 70° or 120° lens helps in good visualisation of antero-lateral aspect, dome of the bladder and in over elevated urethro-vesical junction. Retrograde lenses with an angle of view of more than 90° can visualise the urethra and anterior bladder neck clearly.

Flexible cystoscopes have fibre optic bundles, telescope and irrigating channel combined into a single unit. The greatest advantage is the ability to visualise any aspect of the bladder and urethra, as the camera can be deflected from zero degree to 220°. The tip deflection can be on the same side as the lever deflection or on the opposite side from the lever deflection. The diameter of the flexible cystoscope is usually between 15 and 18 French (Figure 4.2).

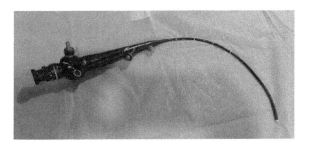

Figure 4.2 Flexible cystoscope.

Comparing the rigid and flexible cystoscopes, the rigid cystoscope has the advantage of better optics, larger lumen for irrigation, in turn giving better visualisation, larger working channels for instruments, and ease of manipulation and orientation. Rigid cystoscopy can be done under local anaesthesia, in the office set-up when it is primarily diagnostic. With the larger diameter rigid scopes, the procedure can be done under general anaesthesia or IV sedation to reduce discomfort. The flexible cystoscope on the other hand, in view of its size, is more comfortable to patients and they are able to tolerate it with just local anaesthetic gel instillation. Flexible cystoscopes are more suitable to be done as an office procedure. In a flexible scope, with the deflection of the tip of the instrument, it is possible to visualise at any angle, the bladder neck, bladder wall, and urethra. Flexible cystoscopy, however, has a longer training curve compared to rigid cystoscopy.

Pre-procedure

Urine analysis with microscopy or a urine culture done about five to seven days before the procedure helps in ruling out a urinary tract infection. An informed consent is obtained prior to the procedure. Antimicrobial prophylaxis is not recommended in routine diagnostic cystoscopy in the absence of risk factors. However, in the presence of risk factors such as, elderly patients, immunodeficiency, long-term steroid use, abnormalities of urinary tract, or in a poorly controlled diabetic, a single dose of aminoglycoside or third generation cephalosporins should suffice for prophylaxis. Prophylaxis lasting less than 24 hours with either a fluoroquinolone or trimethoprim-sulfamethoxazole is recommended for therapeutic procedures.

Indications

Cystoscopy is used mostly as a diagnostic tool in urogynaecological practice. The common diagnostic indications are:

- Haematuria – macroscopic and microscopic
- Bladder pain syndrome (BPS) (chronic pelvic pain, interstitial cystitis)
- Recurrent UTI
- Bladder abnormality on imaging studies
- Abnormal urine cytology
- Voiding abnormalities
- Overactive bladder symptoms, not responding to anticholinergics
- Intra-operative – to check, bladder, urethra, and ureteral integrity, during anti-incontinence procedures and other pelvic surgeries
- In evaluation of anterior vaginal wall cysts
- Evaluation of urinary fistula
- Identification of diverticular opening
- Assessment in cervical cancer, to check bladder involvement
- Bladder mucosal biopsy

Use of cystoscopy as treatment modality is indicated in:

- Insertion and removal of ureteric stents
- Removal of foreign body, calculi, polyp, or tumour in bladder
- Intra-detrusor Botulinum toxin (Botox) injection
- Injection of urethral bulking agents
- Hydrodistension

Contraindication to cystoscopy is active urinary infection. In the presence of pain intolerance, the procedure should not be done as an office procedure and should be done under anaesthesia.

Technique

Patient is placed in the dorsal lithotomy position, with the legs supported and buttocks at the edge of the table. Perineum including the peri-urethral and vagina are prepared. External genitalia and urethral opening visualised prior to cystoscope insertion. Presence of a urethrocele, urethral mucosal prolapse or urethral diverticula is noted. If done under local anaesthesia, 1% lidocaine gel is instilled in the urethra, which acts both as a topical anaesthetic and a lubricant.

A cystoscope is introduced into the urethra under direct vision. A rigid cystoscope is introduced either with or without an obturator and it is usually recommended to introduce it with an obturator in females to minimise urethral trauma. The cystoscope should be directed anteriorly as it enters the urethra in females. At times even with the smallest telescope it might be difficult to negotiate into the urethra and gentle dilatation may be helpful. It is important to avoid forceful dilatation of the urethra.

Cystoscopic examination of urethra and bladder should be systematic. The female urethra is only 2.5–4 cm long. Urethral mucosa should be examined for strictures, diverticular opening, or polyps, and the bladder neck is visualised as scope enters and exits the bladder. Base and trigone of the bladder are initially inspected. Trigone lies proximal to the bladder neck; it is the triangular area bounded by the inter-ureteric ridge and the bladder neck at the base of the bladder. One of the most common features of the trigone is squamous metaplasia, present in up to 50% of the women. It is a benign feature with no malignant potential.

In staging for cervical cancer, when imaging suggests stage 3 or 4 disease, cystoscopy is indicated. The bladder base and trigone appearance such as bullous edema, inflammatory changes, or infiltration has to be documented, and in case of infiltration, biopsy should be part of the evaluation.

Ureteric orifices are slit-like openings easily identifiable by the presence of efflux on either side of the inter-ureteric ridge (Figure 4.3). The ureteral orifices location, number, nature of ureteric efflux (clear, blood stained), and any anatomical distortion is noted. In a woman with anterior vaginal wall prolapse or an underlying cervical mass, identification of trigone or ureteric orifices may be difficult. In such cases, placing a finger inside the vagina and elevating the bladder base with a finger will be helpful.

Blood stained ureteric efflux denotes upper tract pathology and further assessment of the ureter and kidneys is indicated, either by ultrasound or a CT scan of the kidneys, ureters, and bladder (CT KUB). In intra-operative or post-operative

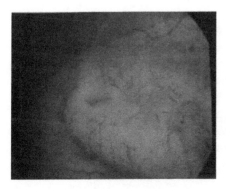 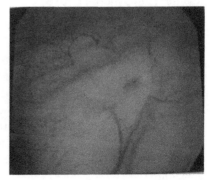

Figure 4.3 Ureteric orifice (right and left sides).

ureteral integrity assessment, presence of just ureteric peristalsis does not rule out ureteral injury. Checking for ureteric efflux after administration of methylthionium chloride or indigo carmine (5 ml) IV is effective in confirming ureteral patency.

Bladder dome is usually identified by the presence of a small air bubble. The surgeon can visualise the lateral walls by rotating the cystoscope and keeping the camera orientation fixed. The dome and posterolateral walls of the bladder are inspected using a 70 or 90° lens on a rigid scope or by retroflection on a flexible scope, right, left, anterior, and posterior. Examination should be thorough, using a reference point like 12 o'clock position and moving the scope either clockwise or anticlockwise from dome towards the bladder neck. The bladder mucosa should be inspected for bladder stones, trabeculations, sacculation, diverticula, mucosal abnormalities, haemorrhagic spots, erythematous patches, papillary/sessile bladder lesions, bladder stones or any foreign body. If a suspicious lesion is identified, it should be biopsied using cystoscopic instruments. Usually, following such biopsies there is no bleeding and there is no need for cauterization.

Bladder diverticulae are herniations of the bladder mucosa between the fibres of the detrusor muscle, which can be congenital or acquired. The acquired variety are secondary to bladder obstruction, associated with trabeculations and commonly present with recurrent urinary tract infection secondary to the stasis in diverticulae. The neck of the diverticular opening can be identified fairly easily on cystoscopy with adequate distension of the bladder. In contrast, urethral diverticular opening identification requires a high index of suspicion and experience.

Identification of fistulous opening in a vesicovaginal fistulae and planning the surgical route and technique, is an essential pre-requisite prior to the fistula repair.

Bladder Pain Syndrome (BPS)

In evaluation of patients with BPS, cystoscopy should be done only under regional or general anaesthesia, because the pain can preclude the assessment of the entire bladder when done under local anaesthetic instillation. The aim of cystoscopy in BPS is to identify classical features of Interstitial cystitis (Figure 4.4). This includes presence of glomerulations, petechial haemorrhages and/or Hunner's Ulcers. However, these typical features are absent in at least 32–42% of patients. The cystoscopy technique in BPS varies in that, at the initial distension the bladder mucosa may not show any abnormality. On double-fill (i.e., refilling after emptying) with hydro-distension, the typical features of interstitial cystitis may become apparent.

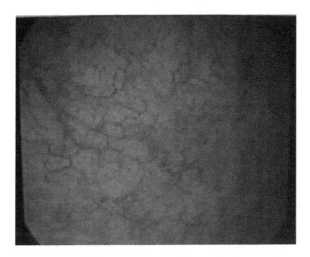

Figure 4.4   Petechial haemorrhagic spots.

Intra-operative Cystoscopy

Identification of intra-operative bladder injury is one of the major indications of cystoscopy. It is an intra-operative step during an incontinence procedure such as mid-urethral slings, pubovaginal slings, Burch colposuspension, and Stamey' procedure. For procedures in which instruments and trocar are introduced via the retropubic space and cystoscopy is done to rule out bladder perforation, certain principles have to be adhered to. The bladder needs to be filled beyond 400 ml and a 70° telescope should be used, as the perforation is likely to be closer to the dome of the bladder and likely to be missed otherwise.

Other pelvic floor surgeries where the risk of bladder or ureteric injury is increased such as in high uterosacral ligament suspension (HUSL) and in other major vaginal and urogynaecological surgeries, the American Urogynaecological Society (AUGS) and the American Urological Society (AUS) recommend cystoscopy. When the risk of ureteric injury is high, administering 5 ml of indigo carmine intravenously, slowly over 5–10 minutes, helps in checking ureteral patency.

In a large series involving 526 patients, routine intraoperative cystoscopy detected 2.9% lower urinary tract injuries in procedures which were not done for incontinence. Anterior colporraphy was the most common cause of unrecognised and unsuspected urinary tract injury, occurring in 2% of anterior vaginal wall repair.

Cystoscopy as Surgical Tool

Hydro-distension using a cystoscope is a simple treatment option in patients with interstitial cystitis. Cystoscopy can be of value in simple procedures such as suprapubic catheterization as an ancillary tool. Insertion and removal of ureteric stents is an ambulatory procedure and can be done with or without imaging guidance.

Cysto-lithotripsy performed by the urologists, in the treatment of bladder calculi is essentially a cystoscopic surgery. Using either a lithotripter or a helium laser, the vesical calculi is broken into smaller fragments and extracted. The procedure can be done as day care but an indwelling catheter may be needed for a couple of days, until the urine clears. Post-operative use of antispasmodic agents helps in the immediate post-operative period.

Use of urethral bulking is one of the treatment options in patients with stress urinary incontinence. Bulking agents such as collagen, macroplastique are injected around the bladder neck under cystoscope guidance. This improves the co-optation of the urethral mucosa and increases the urethral resistance thereby promoting continence.

Intra-detrusor injection of Botulinum toxin is used in the treatment of refractory and neurogenic detrusor overactivity 100 or 200 IU of diluted Onobotulinum toxin A is injected via cystoscope guidance at 20 sites in the detrusor muscle, of 1 ml injections. This is essentially an ambulatory procedure with complications such as urinary tract infection and high post-void residual resolving soon. Though the effect lasts for less than a year, repeat procedures can be done without loss of efficacy.

Side Effects and Complications

Cystoscopy is well tolerated by most patients with the most common side effects being mild burning sensation, urgency, and haematuria. These usually resolve in 24–48 hours. The two most immediate complications of the procedure include bleeding and urinary obstruction, and this should be assessed before the patient leaves the day care centre. Serious complications of cystoscopy such as injury to the urethra or bladder are not common.

Conclusion

Cystoscopy is one of the most important diagnostic tools used by the urologists and urogynaecologists. It is relatively simple and can be performed as an office procedure in most cases. It provides a means of diagnosis for numerous conditions and invaluable intra-operatively in assessing ureteral and bladder integrity. For this reason, it is important for gynaecologists and not just urologists to be trained in this simple procedure.

Further Reading

Foon, R., Elbiss, H., and Moran, P.A. (2006). Cystoscopy for gynaecologists. *Obstet. Gynaecol.* 8: 78–85.

Hanno, P.M., Landis, J.R., Mathews-Cook, Y. et al. (1999). The diagnosis of interstitial cystitis revisited: lessons learned from the National Institutes of Health Interstitial Cystitis Database Study. *J. Urol.* 161: 553–557.

Kwon, C.H., Goldberg, R.P., Koduri, S. et al. (2002). The use of intraoperative cystoscopy in major vaginal and urogynecologic surgeries. *Am. J. Obstet. Gynecol.* 187 (6): 1466–1472.

Ramai, D., Zakhia, K., Etienne, D., and Reddy, M. (2018). Philipp Bozzini (1773–1809): the earliest description of endoscopy. *J. Med. Biogr* 26 (2): 137–141.

Weinberger, M.W. (1998). Cystourethroscopy for the practicing gynaecologist. *Clin. Obstet. Gynecol.* 41: 764–766.

5

Role of Nurse Practitioners in Ambulatory Urogynaecological Care

Angie Rantell

Introduction

Ambulatory care is defined as 'a personal healthcare consultation including diagnosis, observation, treatment, intervention, and rehabilitation services using advanced medical technology or procedures delivered on an outpatient basis (i.e. where the patient's stay at the hospital or clinic, from the time of registration to discharge, occurs on a single calendar day).' Many different specialties across healthcare settings provide ambulatory care services, and they represent the most significant contributors to increasing hospital expenditures to set-up services whilst improving the performance of the healthcare system in most countries, including most developing countries. Ambulatory gynaecology services were first reported in the literature in 2005, and many healthcare organisations around the world are actively moving towards an ambulatory model of care because it has been found to be associated with reduced morbidity and cost savings.

In some health systems, urinary incontinence has traditionally been seen solely as a nursing problem. The evolution of the nursing role and the provision of ambulatory care has significantly improved care and available treatment options. The role of the nurse practitioner (NP) was first developed in the United Kingdom (UK) in the 1980s and they now play a fundamental clinical role in many specialties, especially continence.

This chapter aims to describe the role of the NP within an ambulatory urogynaecology setting. It will discuss the different facets of the NP role prior to suggesting examples of diagnostics and treatments that can be provided by an NP as well as reviewing the additional risk and governance structures that need to be in place for safe working.

Ambulatory Urology and Urogynaecology, First Edition. Edited by Abhay Rane and Ajay Rane.
© 2021 John Wiley & Sons Ltd. Published 2021 by John Wiley & Sons Ltd.

Who is a Nurse Practitioner (NP)?

The traditional nursing role is similar throughout the world and generally involves patient observations, toileting, personal hygiene assistance, medication administration, wound care, post-operative care, and specific tasks assigned to them by the doctors in charge of the patient's care. In many countries, however, this role has evolved not only as a result of reduced working hours for doctors and increasing demands for health services, but also due to enhanced education for nurses. NPs not only provide advanced clinical care but are also involved in research, audit, education-and-policy development, and they have an organisational role, as part of management teams; they may also be responsible for budgets, purchasing, and finding suppliers.

From a clinical perspective NPs work autonomously, providing general and specialist health assessment, diagnostic investigations and treatment planning, as well as performing certain treatments. Many will be independent nurse prescribers. Ultimately, NPs in specialist practice are exercising higher levels of judgement, discretion, and decision-making in clinical care. A significant part of the role is also in the education and counselling of patients regarding their condition, prognosis, and available treatments, in addition to being a patient advocate.

One of the expanding roles of all NPs has been in the performance of minor surgery. It was reported by Dunlop in 2010 that in several specialties, nurses have started to undertake minor surgical procedures to ease waiting-list pressures and to increase capacity to enable training of more junior doctors in complex cases. This has included performing procedures such as flexible cystoscopy hysteroscopy, insertion of supra-pubic catheters and intra-detrusor injections of botulinum toxin A under local anaesthetic or mild sedation. With the advent of more surgical devices for incontinence that can be inserted under local anaesthetic this role may soon expand further. NPs have been shown to be as effective as junior doctors at many of these procedures. A Cochrane Review also explored the substitution of doctors with NPs and found similar patient health outcomes, at least in the short-term, over the range of care investigated. Within a continence/urogynaecology setting, the role of the NP has been reported as essential for service development, to ensure integrated care and optimal continence care packages.

To perform this role, NPs must have an advanced level of understanding of anatomy and physiology, be experienced and proficient clinical decision makers. A formal assessment pathway to ensure competency must be performed by an appropriate medical professional to ensure safe practice in line with regulatory bodies and individual trust/hospital protocols.

Table 5.1 Potential diagnostics and treatments.

	Urogynaecology
Diagnostics:	*Treatment/Procedures:*
Uroflowmetry	Pelvic floor muscle training
Filling & voiding cystometry	Bladder retraining
Video cysto-urethrography	Bladder instillations
Ambulatory urodynamics monitoring	Posterior tibial nerve stimulation
Abdominal/pelvic ultrasound	Vaginal pessaries for prolapse and incontinence
Pelvic floor ultrasound	Trial without catheter/ trial of void
Flexible/rigid cystoscopy	Supra-pubic catheter changes
	Ureteric stent removal
	Botulinum toxin A injection
	Injection of bulking agents
	Mini-slings
	Laser therapy
	Perineal wound care
	Telephone follow-up for post-op women

What Can a Urogynaecology Nurse Practitioner Do?

Within the ambulatory setting, a vast array of assessments and procedures can be performed by a specialist urogynaecology NP. These may be related to more traditional nursing care roles or advanced diagnostics/treatments within urogynaecology, general gynaecology, or early pregnancy care. Table 5.1 lists some of the assessments and procedures that NPs perform in relation to urogynaecology.

Educational/Training Requirements

There is considerable international variation with the level of education required for NPs. Generally, most have a minimum of a bachelor's degree, but other posts require a minimum of a master's degree or even a PhD. All NPs will have to demonstrate a minimum number of years of clinical experience within their field and evidence of post-graduate education. There are currently no educational courses dedicated to urogynaecology, however, educational courses on continence and also in gynaecology are available for nurses in the UK, the United States, Europe, and Australia. More courses are beginning to appear in Asia, notably Hong Kong and Singapore.

For many ambulatory procedures there are national training requirements. For example, in the UK, the British Association of Urology (BAUS) and the British Association of Urology Nurses (BAUN) have a training guideline for nurse cystoscopists, including stent removal, Botox injections and biopsies/diathermy. These should be used where available to encourage safe working practice. In many countries, it is necessary to provide proof of training and perform re-validation for professional indemnity.

The main challenge for NPs and for the medics training them is in the time taken and number of procedures that need to be performed to ensure competency. This is generally far more extensive than the training requirements for junior doctors but is essential to fulfil the increased requirements for governance and safety.

Documentation

Accurate documentation is a fundamental part of healthcare and needs to be adapted for use by NPs in specialist services to ensure that it meets the governance requirements. If the ambulatory service is predominantly led by NPs, an operational policy should be developed to incorporate all clinical and potential emergency scenarios. Appropriate plans should be in place for discussing patients with a multidisciplinary team (MDT) and for onward referral if appropriate. The policy should act as a guide for all staff working within the service and for those referring patients to the service. Treatment protocols should also be available to guide all clinical staff performing or assisting in procedures, to ensure exactly what their responsibilities are and that appropriate training is provided.

Table 5.2 shows criteria to be included in an operational policy and treatment protocol.

For many services, it is a requirement that NPs use pre-approved procedure-specific consent forms and patient information leaflets. These should be approved by the local governance committee to ensure that they are accurate, at a reading age appropriate for the local population, and clearly outline whether the procedure will be performed by an NP or a doctor. Depending on the healthcare service, it may be necessary to have these available in a range of languages.

In line with the recommendations of the World Health Organisation, a safer surgical checklist should also be completed before all procedures and, if indicated, a decontamination audit trail should also be recorded regardless of the professional performing the procedure.

Table 5.2 Criteria for operational policy and treatment protocol.

Operational Policy	Treatment Protocol
Overview of service	Indications/contra-indications
Location	for procedure
Hours of operations	Potential complications
Medical/nursing establishment	Consent and accountability
Internal/External referral pathways	Key points
Admission/Discharge criteria	Patient preparation
Transfer to inpatient care	Equipment
Follow-up	Performing the procedure
Supplies and procurement	Post-procedure
Cleaning and maintenance	Follow-up
Performance, monitoring, management and audit	Documentation

Managing Risks and Governance Requirements

For many services, the delay or concern of moving towards NP-led ambulatory services has been around legislative issues, lack of understanding about how the nursing role can be advanced, lack of supervision, and administrative restrictions. Although NPs work in an autonomous role, they must have access to an MDT to discuss complex cases and findings. The ability to capture still pictures or live videos can prevent diagnostics having to be repeated, in addition to aiding discussion and further treatment planning with the wider team.

A further concern is the management of emergency situations or complications associated with certain treatments. NPs should, as a minimum, be trained in basic life support to ensure that any intra-procedure emergencies can be managed appropriately. The level of experience, training, and supervision will dictate how they manage complications, and this should be included as part of NPs' education. Regular audits of practice, safety, and outcomes should be performed to ensure that they are in line with expectations.

Conclusions

NPs have a lot to offer towards ambulatory service models of care. Although there is a lack of data specifically regarding urogynaecology, the NP role has been shown to improve patient care, reduce medical workload, improve waiting times, and, following an initial training period, be cost-effective in the long-term. With a receptive medical team that is willing to provide training and indirect supervision, the role can continue to expand and evolve along with clinical practice.

Further Reading

Berman P. Organization of ambulatory care provision: a critical determinant of health system performance in developing countries. *Bulletin of the World Health Organization* 2000; 78 (6):791.

Dunlop, N., 2010. Advancing the role of minor surgery for nurses. *British Journal of Nursing*, 19 (11), pp. 685–691.

Geurts-Laurent MG, Reeves D, Hermens RP, Braspenning JC, Grol RP, Sibbald BS. Substitution of doctors by nurses in primary care. *Cochrane Database of Systematic Reviews* 2004; 4: CD001271, doi: https://doi.org/10.1002/14651858. CD001271.pub2.

Ghoshal, S. and Smith, AR., 2005. Ambulatory surgery in urogynaecology. *Best Practice & Research. Clinical Obstetrics & Gynaecology*, 19 (5), pp. 769–777

Hudson, L. (2005). Best practice in care planning and documentation. In: *Nurse Led Continence Clinics* (ed. R. Addison). Coloplast, UK: Peterborough.

Winston, W.J. (1985). *Marketing Ambulatory Care Services*, 9–11. UK: Routledge: Abingdon-on-Thames.

6

Non-Surgical Management of Pelvic Floor Disorders

Arjunan Tamilselvi

Pelvic floor disorders of urinary incontinence, pelvic organ prolapse (POP) and anal dysfunction have the potential to significantly affect the quality of life (QoL). All these conditions are amenable to non-surgical management and their efficacy has been studied in detail. Conservative measures of lifestyle changes, pelvic floor exercises (PFE), use of pessaries, and pharmacological interventions play a major role, either as a short-term intervention or as a definitive treatment in pelvic floor disorders.

General Life-Style Interventions

Elements of general life-style interventions of exercise, weight loss, smoking cessation, and avoiding constipation are all commonly applied in the management of pelvic floor disorders. The advantage of these interventions is that, they can be started solely based on the clinical history, without any exhaustive diagnostic work-up.

Weight loss in women who are overweight or obese has been shown to improve the symptoms of urinary and faecal incontinence. One study has shown in obese women, who lost 3–5% of their baseline weight, there was a 47% reduction in stress incontinence episodes. With weight loss surgeries, improvement in urinary and faecal incontinence symptoms has been demonstrated.

In patients with POP, studies have shown that risk of prolapse progression increases in overweight and obese women compared to women with healthy body mass index and this progression was demonstrated consistently in all three compartments, anterior, apical, and posterior. However, weight loss has not been

Ambulatory Urology and Urogynaecology, First Edition. Edited by Abhay Rane and Ajay Rane.
© 2021 John Wiley & Sons Ltd. Published 2021 by John Wiley & Sons Ltd.

shown to improve prolapse symptoms and not associated with reduction in the grading of prolapse. The progression with increased BMI and the lack of regression with weight loss, suggests that damage to pelvic floor with obesity, might become irreversible over time.

Smoking is associated with chronic cough and bronchitis, which can increase intra-abdominal pressure and thereby weaken the pelvic floor muscle and connective tissue. Epidemiological studies have shown a strong association between urinary and anal incontinence and smoking. There are no studies to demonstrate that smoking cessation reduces the progression of urinary incontinence, overactive bladder symptom (OAB) and anal incontinence. The association between smoking and POP appears to be variable.

Pelvic Floor Exercises

Pelvic floor exercises (PFE) or pelvic floor muscle training (PFMT) have shown to be an important component in the treatment of pelvic floor disorders. Commonly referred to as Kegel's exercise, it has been in practice since 1948. In PFMT, the pelvic floor muscles are assessed and regular contraction of the pelvic floor muscles is taught to improve the strength and endurance of muscles and thereby facilitate better support of the pelvic organs. Assessment of pelvic floor muscle involves vaginal palpation of the muscle to assess its strength and tone. The Modified Oxford grading system is widely used to quantify muscle strength (Table 6.1). PFMT, when done correctly, is likely to increase the pelvic muscle strength and thereby the levator plate.

In both urinary and faecal incontinence, PFMT is used as first-line intervention with or without behavioural approaches. In urinary incontinence, PFMT is more commonly employed in patients with stress urinary incontinence (SUI) and less commonly in those with urge or mixed incontinence. In a Cochrane review (2018),

Table 6.1 Modified Oxford scale.

Modified Oxford Grading for Pelvic Floor Muscles	
0	No contraction/muscle activity
1	Minor muscle flicker
2	Weak muscle activity with no circular contraction
3	Moderate muscle contraction
4	Good muscle contraction
5	Strong muscle contraction

the cure rate for SUI with PFMT was 56% compared to 6% in the control group. The review also showed reduction in the number of leakage episodes and improvement in urinary incontinence specific to QoL, all reiterating the beneficial effect of PFMT in SUI.

PFMT and biofeedback have been shown to alleviate the symptoms of faecal incontinence. Compared to urinary incontinence, however, the data on PFMT in faecal incontinence management is limited. Biofeedback, is a way of notifying the patient when certain physiological events are occurring. Using an anorectal manometry or surface electromyography (EMG), biofeedback therapy focuses on rectal sensitivity training, strength training using visual or auditory signals for proper muscle isolation and coordination training focusing on rectal distension and anal sphincter contraction. The success rate for PFMT combined with biofeedback in faecal incontinence varies from 38 to 100%.

The efficacy of PFE in the treatment of POP was evaluated in the multicentre randomised controlled POPPY trial (pelvic organ prolapse physiotherapy trial). The study evaluated whether one-to-one PFMT would reduce the symptoms of prolapse and the need for further treatment in women with stage I–III prolapse. There was a good improvement of prolapse symptoms and reduction in its severity, in women doing PFMT compared to the controls, but there was no statistically significant difference in the objective improvement of POP assessed by pelvic organ prolapse quantification staging (POP-Q). Nevertheless, since treatment for POP is used to alleviate the POP symptoms, PFE remains the first mode of intervention in patients with POP.

Supervised PFMT and Biofeedback

PFMT though being a simple exercise, about a third doing Kegel's exercise do not contract the pelvic muscles and instead contract the lower abdominal, thigh or buttock muscles. Learning the correct technique is an important aspect in the success of PFMT. The first step is to identify the pelvic floor muscle and several techniques are taught, such as pretending to trying to avoid passing gas or trying to stop urine flow in mid-stream. Once the correct muscles are identified, the PFE is initially practised in the lying position and thereafter can be done in sitting or standing position. The minimum number of contractions recommended is 30 per day, spread out throughout the day. Women receiving regular and frequent supervised PFMT with a health professional, are more likely to show improvement of their symptoms than women doing training with little or no supervision. The most intensive programmes in terms of supervision, weekly over three months, are shown to be the most successful.

In an attempt to improve the efficacy of PFMT, it has been evaluated using other modalities as adjunct, such as vaginal cones, electrical stimulation, and use of magnetic chairs. Vaginal cones of increasing weight, in equal shape and volume are used. Starting with the lightest weight, gradually increasing the cone weight successively, women are taught to place the cone into the vagina while standing and hold it in place with voluntary contraction of the pelvic floor. The heaviest weight that can be retained by the women is called the active cone and women are advised to exercise the pelvic floor muscle using this. This effectively acts like a biofeedback helping in the PFMT.

Electrical stimulation is a more sophisticated form of biofeedback therapy in PFMT. Electrodes are inserted into the middle third of the vagina and using an on–off pulse cycle, over a range of 0–100 mA, the maximum current intensity comfortably tolerated by the patient is delivered. A study comparing PFE, use of vaginal cones, and electrical stimulation identified all three interventions as equally effective in women with urinary incontinence. Use of cones and electrical stimulation did not significantly increase the strength of pelvic floor muscle as compared to PFMT alone.

Use of magnetic chair was introduced as an additional tool in the conservative management of urinary incontinence. The patient sits in a specially designed chair and within the seat is a magnetic field generator, that delivers rapidly changing magnetic impulse. The principle is that magnetic impulse delivered to the pelvic floor can increase its muscle strength. The studies have not shown any significant improvement of symptoms of both urinary and faecal incontinence with extracorporeal magnetic stimulation.

PFMT has been shown to be an effective strategy in patients with SUI, faecal incontinence, and in a group of patients with stage I–III POP. Hence, it would be the first line of conservative management, and vaginal cones, electrical stimulation, and extracorporeal magnetic stimulation can be offered to women who find it difficult to identify and contract their pelvic floor.

Bladder Re-training

In patients with urge incontinence, behavioural interventions such as bladder training with patient education on type and amount of fluid intake – based on the bladder diary – scheduled voiding, and urge-suppression strategies constitute the first line of intervention. This is often reinforced with PFMT and biofeedback. The PFE can increase the bladder outlet resistance and is also thought to inhibit spontaneous bladder contractions, resulting in reduced leakage. In patients with OAB, bladder training is an important strategy in reducing the urge episodes. The aim is to increase the time interval between voids to three hours. Patients are asked to start with shorter intervals and gradually increase the time interval using urge-suppression strategies such as crossing legs or contracting pelvic floor muscles, until the three-hour interval is achieved. Restricting alcohol, caffeine, and aerated drinks and ensuring last fluid intake is at least one to two hours before bedtime are other measures helpful in OAB.

Pessaries

Pessaries are commonly employed as non-surgical treatment option in women with prolapse. A pessary is a vaginal support device made of inert material such as silicone or plastic and can be used to treat symptoms of POP and SUI. A variety of pessaries are available, broadly classified into support pessaries, space-filling pessaries, and incontinence pessaries (Figures 6.1–6.7). The most common types of

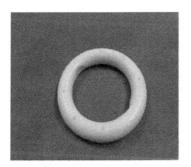

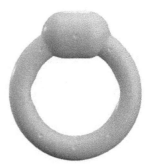

Figure 6.1 Ring pessary without knob and with knob.

Figure 6.2 Dish pessary with knob.

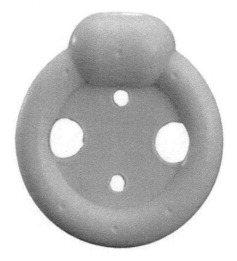

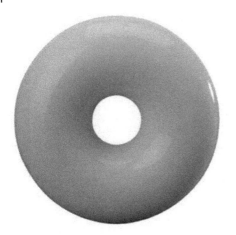

Figure 6.3   Doughnut pessary.

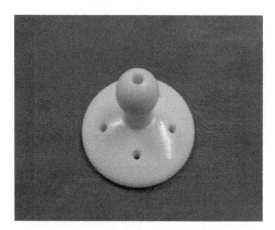

Figure 6.4   Gellhorn pessary.

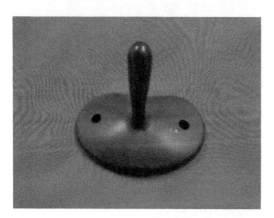

Figure 6.5   Shelf pessary.

Figure 6.6 Cube pessary.

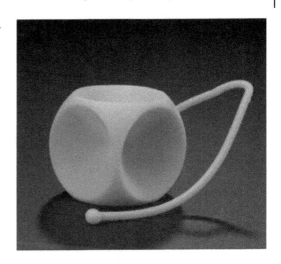

Figure 6.7 Inflatoball pessary.

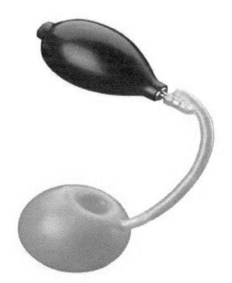

pessaries in clinical use are the ring pessary and the Gellhorn pessary. The incontinence pessaries have the addition of a knob that can fit against the bladder neck, thereby preventing a urine leak.

The commonest group in which a pessary is used for POP are, the elderly frail patients, with or without co-morbid problems which preclude surgery. In young women, pessaries are used for POP and SUI in those who prefer conservative management rather than surgery.

Choice of the pessary depends on the presenting problem, stage of prolapse, and the desire for sexual activity. In patients presenting with POP and SUI, the incontinence pessaries can provide support to pelvic organs and to the bladder neck. The selection between space-occupying and support pessary is largely dependent on the sexual history of the women. Space-filling pessaries cannot be used in patients who are sexually active, unless they can be trained on self-insertion and removal technique. Most clinicians will avoid inserting pessaries that pose difficulty with insertion and removal, particularly in the elderly.

Prior to fitting the pessary, a pelvic examination should assess the width and length of vagina, stage and compartment of prolapse, presence of infection, ulceration, or atrophic changes. Topical oestrogen cream can be prescribed over two to four-week period prior to insertion in those with significant atrophic changes. Pessary treatment should aim to relieve the prolapse symptom. Appropriate size and type of pessary should be selected, to avoid pain and ulceration of vaginal mucosa. Pessary fitting is an art rather than science.

Pessaries are sometimes used to see what would be the effect of surgery for POP on urinary symptoms, especially in advanced stages of POP. This is called a 'pessary trial'. If any occult SUI is revealed with pessary prior to surgery, procedure to correct SUI can be combined along with prolapse surgery.

The overall success rate for prolapse symptoms with pessaries is quoted around 71%. The PESsary Symptom Relief Impact (PESSRI) study, looked at the symptom relief outcomes using standardized questionnaires, with randomised crossover trial of the ring with support and Gellhorn pessary. The study showed there were statistically and clinically significant improvements in the majority of pelvic floor distress inventory (PFDI) and pelvic floor impact questionnaire (PFIQ) scoring with both pessaries and no clinically significant differences between the two. Both effectively relieved the symptoms of protrusion and voiding problem. In patients with SUI, ring pessaries with and without support were found to be effective in relieving symptoms in 78% and 63%, respectively, in a study. The success rates with pessaries have been quoted from 41 to 74% in different studies, irrespective of the compartment of prolapse. A long or wide vagina is not a contraindication for vaginal pessary. If pessary fitting is successful at the end of four weeks, most women would continue to use it over five years. The usual recommendation for pessary change is every three to four months, and at each change the vaginal wall should be examined to rule out ulceration.

There are very few complications associated with pessaries and they include discharge, pain, discomfort, ulceration, bleeding, constipation, and rarely disimpaction. When using in the elderly age group, the social situation should be addressed to check if patient has support system in place for regular pessary change.

Pessaries are contraindicated in the presence of cervical or vaginal ulcerations, undiagnosed vaginal bleeding, active pelvic infection, and patients allergic to silicone or latex.

Pharmacotherapy

In women with urinary incontinence, the role of pharmacotherapy in patients with OAB is well defined compared to those with SUI. In the broadest definition, SUI is the result of urethral sphincter incompetence and pathologically results from urethral or bladder neck hypermobility or reduced mucosal co-optation in intrinsic sphincter deficiency.

Alpha-adrenoceptor (α-AR) agonists, estrogens, and tricyclic antidepressants (TCAs) have been used in the pharmacological treatment of SUI. There is little or no evidence of the effectiveness of these drugs, and some of them have been shown to have significant adverse effects. Alpha agonists can cause a rise in blood pressure, and imipramine can cause orthostatic hypotension and constipation. Oestrogen deficiency is identified as a causative factor for SUI, but oestrogen therapy is more effective in patients with urge incontinence and its role in SUI is controversial. Duloxetine, a serotonin nor-adrenaline re-uptake inhibitor (SNRI) has been used in the treatment of SUI. This drug has shown moderate efficacy in the treatment of mild to moderate SUI with adverse events of nausea, constipation, dry mouth, and fatigue limiting its use.

In patients with OAB symptoms, with or without urge urinary incontinence (UUI), the primary modality of intervention along with life style intervention is pharmacotherapy. Urgency, frequency, nocturia, and urge incontinence result from detrusor contractions during the storage phase of the micturition cycle. The contraction is predominantly mediated by the muscarinic receptors on the detrusor muscle, so anticholinergic (antimuscarinic) drugs are the medications of choice in OAB. The new entrant in the pharmacotherapy for OAB is the β3-adrenoceptor agonist, Mirabegron. The mode of action is by stimulation of the β3-adrenoceptors on the detrusor muscle, promoting bladder relaxation during the storage phase.

The different anticholinergic drugs, oxybutynin, tolterodine, trospium chloride, solifenacin, darifenacin, fesoterodine are all associated with systemic anticholinergic effects of dry mouth and constipation with varying incidence. Oxybutynin the non-selective anticholinergic, also exerts muscle relaxant and local anaesthetic effects. Tolterodine, trospium, solifenacin, darifenacin, and fesoterodine are selective antimuscarinic agents, acting on the M2 and M3 receptors. The very low penetration of darifenacin, across the blood brain barrier is beneficial in the elderly, as it is less likely to cause confusion.

The Cochrane systematic review in 2012, compared the anticholinergic drugs against each other. In terms of efficacy, all these anticholinergic drugs have been shown to be effective, with reduction in urgency and incontinence episodes. The systematic review comparing the oral immediate release (IR) oxybutynin and tolterodine, concluded the latter might be preferred with a reduced risk of dry mouth. The extended-release preparations are preferred to the IR because of lesser-side-effect profile. Solifenacin, and fesoterodine when compared to IR tolterodine, the former two have lesser incidence of dry mouth and constipation. Because the efficacy is similar for the antimuscarinics, it is the side-effect profile, that determines the continuation of treatment.

Mirabegron, a β3-adrenoceptor agonist with its different receptor target, should not have the anticholinergic side-effect profile. The efficacy of mirabegron in the treatment of OAB has been demonstrated in randomised, placebo-controlled trials. The drug has been efficacious in reducing the mean number of micturition and incontinence episodes per 24 hours, as well as in improving other secondary outcomes such as OAB symptoms and QoL measures.

Common adverse drug events seen with mirabegron include hypertension, nasopharyngitis, urinary tract infections, and headache. Given the efficacy and safety data currently available, mirabegron represents a reasonable alternative to antimuscarinics for patients with OAB.

Percutaneous Posterior Tibial Nerve Stimulation (PTNS)

Percutaneous posterior tibial nerve stimulation (PTNS) is a neuromodulation technique, where the sacral nerve plexus is indirectly stimulated and the detrusor and rectal function/activity is modified. The mechanism of neuromodulation is not completely understood, and alteration of the afferent and efferent pathways between the brain, brain stem, and pelvic organs are thought to modulate the voiding reflex and facilitate storage. PTNS is a treatment option in women with refractory OAB, who do not respond to pharmacotherapy and in those with urge faecal incontinence.

The sympathetic and parasympathetic innervation of the pelvic organs is mediated via nerves originating from L2 to S4 segments of the spinal cord. The sciatic nerve is composed of fibres from L4 to S3 and one of its branches is the posterior tibial nerve. Stimulation of this peripheral nerve is believed to cause cross-signalling between the sympathetic and parasympathetic postganglionic nerve terminals and synapses, and is postulated to modulate neural transmission altering bladder and rectal function.

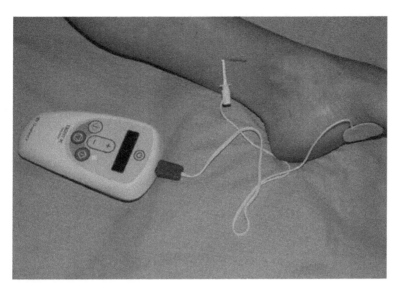

Figure 6.8 PTNS connection.

PTNS involves insertion of a 34-gauge needle approximately three fingers breadth cephalad to the medial malleolus, between the posterior margin of the tibia and soleus muscle. The tip of the needle should be close to the posterior tibial nerve without actually touching it. The needle is inserted to a depth of about 2–4 cm at an angulation of 60–90° and the adhesive electrode is fixed near the arch of the foot (Figure 6.8). The needle and the electrode are connected to a low voltage (9 V) stimulator with an adjustable pulse intensity of 0–10 mA, a fixed pulse width of 200 microseconds and a frequency of 20 Hz.

During the initial test stimulation, the amplitude is slowly increased until the large toe starts to curl or the toes start to fan. Once optimal position is assured, stimulation is applied at an intensity level well tolerated by the patient and can be increased or decreased during the treatment. During PTNS, the patient's leg is comfortably elevated and supported. Most treatment schedules consist of 12 outpatient consecutive treatment sessions lasting 30 minutes each, given 1–2 times/week.

The overall subjective success, defined as improved QoL or willingness to continue treatment, was found in 56–63% of OAB patients. Overall objective success with ≥50% decrease in urge or UUI and 25% reduction in daytime and/or night time frequency was found in 33–71%. In those with faecal incontinence, PTNS has shown statistically significant improvement in patients with urge and mixed faecal incontinence, with improvement in the Cleveland Clinic Florida (CCF)-FI score, with an associated improvement in the QoL score. Studies have also shown significant improvements in the median deferment time and median number of weekly faecal incontinence episodes.

PTNS is a low risk non-surgical treatment option with limited contraindications. It should not be used in those under the age of 18, patients with pacemakers or implantable defibrillators, coagulopathy, neuropathy, those who are currently pregnant or with the intention to become pregnant, and in those with local skin pathology. Apart from the other conservative measures employed in pelvic floor disorders, PTNS is the other intervention most suitable to be done in the ambulatory setting.

Conclusion

In POP and SUI, surgical management though an effective intervention – it might not be the treatment of choice in some women. PFMT and pessaries are a good first line option in those women, and in those with OAB, PFE, bladder retraining combined with pharmacotherapy are the treatment of choice for the majority.

Further Reading

Cundiff, G.W., Amundsen, C.L., Bent, A.E. et al. (2007). The PESSRI study: symptom relief outcomes of a randomized crossover trial of the ring and Gellhorn pessaries. *American Journal of Obstetrics and Gynecology* 196 (4): 405.e1–405.e8.

Dumoulin, C., Cacciari, L.P., and Hay-Smith, E.J.C. (2018). Pelvic floor muscle training versus no treatment, or inactive control treatments, for urinary incontinence in women. *Cochrane Database of Systematic Reviews* (10): CD005654. https://doi.org/10.1002/14651858.CD005654.pub4.

Hagen, S., Stark, D., Glazener, C. et al. (2013). Individualised pelvic floor muscle training in women with pelvic organ prolapse (POPPY): a multicentre randomised controlled trial. *Lancet* 383: 796–806.

Madhuvrata, P., Cody, J.D., Ellis, G. et al. (2012). Which anticholinergic drug for overactive bladder symptoms in adults. *Cochrane Database of Systematic Reviews* (1): CD005429. https://doi.org/10.1002/14651858.CD005429.pub2.

7

Ambulatory Surgical Procedures in Stress Urinary Incontinence

Dudley Robinson

Introduction

The term stress urinary incontinence (SUI) may be used to describe the symptom or sign of urinary leakage on coughing or exertion but should not be regarded as a diagnosis. A diagnosis of urodynamic stress incontinence (USI) can only be made after urodynamic investigation, and this is defined as the involuntary leakage of urine during increased abdominal pressure in the absence of a detrusor contraction.

All women who complain of the symptom of SUI will initially benefit from lifestyle advice and pelvic floor muscle training (PFMT). Those who fail to improve with conservative measures may benefit from Duloxetine or may ultimately require continence surgery. This chapter will focus on those surgical options that may be performed as ambulatory or outpatient procedures.

Epidemiology

Stress incontinence is the most commonly reported type of urinary incontinence in women. In a large epidemiological study of 27 936 women from Norway, 25% of women reported urinary incontinence of whom 7% considered it to be significant. The prevalence of incontinence increased with age. When considering the type of incontinence, 50% of women complained of stress, 11% of urge, and 36% of mixed incontinence. The prevalence of urinary incontinence among nulliparous women ranged from 8 to 32% and increased with age. In general, parity was associated

Ambulatory Urology and Urogynaecology, First Edition. Edited by Abhay Rane and Ajay Rane.
© 2021 John Wiley & Sons Ltd. Published 2021 by John Wiley & Sons Ltd.

with incontinence and the first delivery was the most significant factor. In the age group 20–34 years, the relative risk of stress incontinence was 2.7 (95% CI: 2.0–3.5) for primiparous women and 4.0 (95% CI: 2.5–6.4) for multiparous women. There was a similar association for mixed incontinence, although, not for urge incontinence.

Pathophysiology

There are various underlying causes that result in weakness of one or more of the components of the urethral sphincter mechanism (Table 7.1).

The bladder neck and proximal urethra are normally situated in an intra-abdominal position above the pelvic floor and are supported by the pubo-urethral ligaments. Damage to either the pelvic floor musculature (levator ani) or pubo-urethral ligaments may result in descent of the proximal urethra such that it is no

Table 7.1 Causes of stress urinary incontinence.

Urethral hypermobility
Urogenital prolapse
Pelvic floor damage or denervation
Parturition
Pelvic surgery
Menopause
Urethral scarring
Vaginal (urethral) surgery
Incontinence surgery
Urethral dilatation or urethrotomy
Recurrent urinary tract infections
Radiotherapy
Raised intra-abdominal pressure
Pregnancy
Chronic cough (bronchitis)
Abdominal/pelvic mass
Faecal impaction
Ascites
(Obesity)

longer an intra-abdominal organ and this results in leakage of urine per urethra during stress.

This theory has given rise to the concept of the 'hammock hypothesis,' which suggests that the posterior position of the vagina provides a backboard against which increasing intra-abdominal forces compress the urethra. This is supported by the fact that continent women experience an increase in intra-urethral closure pressure during coughing. This pressure rise is lost in women with stress incontinence, although, may be restored following successful continence surgery.

In addition to pelvic floor damage, there is also evidence to suggest that stress incontinence may be caused by primary urethral sphincter weakness or intrinsic sphincter deficiency (ISD). In order to distinguish this type of stress incontinence from that caused by descent and rotation of the bladder neck during straining, the Blaivis Classification has been described based on video-cystourethrography observations. This proposes that Type I and Type II stress incontinence are caused principally by urethral hypermobility, whereas Type III, or ISD, is caused by a primary weakness in the urethral sphincter. Factors associated with ISD are pudendal denervation injuries, loss of integrity of the striated urethral sphincter and urethral smooth muscle, as well as the loss of urethral mucosa and submucosal urethral cushions.

The 'mid-urethral theory' or 'integral theory' described by Petros and Ulmsten is based on earlier studies suggesting that the distal and mid-urethra play an important role in the continence mechanism and that the maximal urethral closure pressure is at the mid urethral point. This theory proposes that damage to the pubourethral ligaments supporting the urethra, impaired support of the anterior vaginal wall to the mid urethra and weakened function of part of the pubococcygeal muscles, which insert adjacent to the urethra, are responsible for causing stress incontinence.

Ambulatory Procedures for Stress Urinary Incontinence

The acceptance of the 'Integral Theory' of incontinence and the success of mid-urethral sling surgery has transformed the approach to continence surgery. There has been a shift from more traditional procedures such as colposuspension and autologous fascial slings, which required an in-patient stay, to day-case procedures. Minimally invasive surgery is associated with less morbidity and considerable cost savings. This had led to a move towards minimally invasive procedures performed as a day-care procedure in an ambulatory setting (Table 7.2).

Table 7.2 Ambulatory procedures for stress urinary incontinence.

Urethral Bulking Agents

Single Incision Mini-Slings

Laser Therapy

Radiofrequency Ablation

Urethral Bulking Agents

Urethral bulking agents may be performed in the ambulatory clinic under local anaesthetic. They are particularly useful in younger women who haven't yet completed their families, in the elderly with co-morbidities, and in those women, who have undergone previous operations and have demonstrated ISD.

Although the actual substance that is injected may differ, the principle is the same. It is injected either periurethrally or transurethrally on either side of the bladder neck or mid-urethra under cystoscopic control. It is intended to increase urethral coaptation without causing out-flow obstruction.

There are now a number of different products available (Table 7.3). The use of minimally invasive implantation systems has also allowed some of these procedures to be performed in the ambulatory setting without the need for concomitant cystoscopy.

Table 7.3 Urethral bulking agents.

Urethral Bulking Agent	Application Technique
Polydimethylsiloxane **(Macroplastique)**	Cystoscopic Implantation System
Pyrolytic carbon coated zirconium oxide beads **(Durasphere)**	Cystoscopic
Calcium Hydroxylapatite in carboxymethylcellulose gel **(Coaptite)**	Cystoscopic
Polyacrylamide hydrogel **(Bulkamid)**	Cystoscopic
Vinyl Dimethyl Polydimethylsiloxane (PDMS) Polymer **(Urolastic)**	Implantation System
Polycaprolactone (PCL) **(Urolon)**	Cystoscopic

Macroplastique

Macroplastique (Cogentix) (Figure 7.1) is a particulate bulking agent composed of polydimethylsiloxane particles suspended in a bio-excretable carrier gel that is removed un-metabolised by renal excretion within one week. The carrier gel is then, over time, replaced by host collagen. Macroplastique may be injected using a cystoscopic approach, a periurethral approach, or by using the Macroplastique implantation system (MIS).

As with most bulking agents Macroplastique was compared to the Contigen Collagen Implant (Bard) in a large North American study of 248 women with USI. The outcome was assessed objectively using pad tests and subjectively at 12 months. Overall, the objective cure and improvement rates favoured Macroplastique over Contigen (74 vs 65%; p = 0.13). Although this difference was not statistically significant, subjective cure rates were higher in the Macroplastique group (41 vs 29%; p = 0.07).

Macroplastique is one of the few bulking agents to have long-term efficacy data with dry rates of 67% reported at one year and 41% at two years, as well as 85% improvement rates at two years. These results are supported by a systematic review and meta-analysis of 958 patients from 23 studies, which demonstrated 75% (95%CI: 69–81) in the short term, 73% (95%CI: 62–83) in the mid-term and

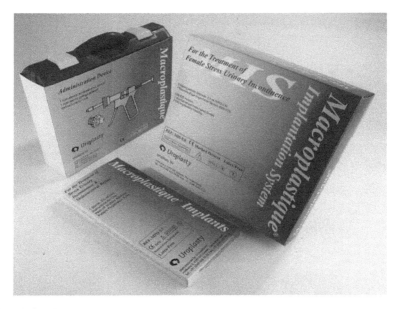

Figure 7.1 Macroplastique.

64% (95%CI: 57–71) in the longer term. Dry rates were 43% (95%CI: 33–54), 37% (95%CI: 28–46) and 36% (95%CI: 69–81), respectively. Importantly, there were no serious adverse events reported.

Bulkamid

Bulkamid (Contura) (Figure 7.2) is a homogenous biocompatible bulking agent composed of non-degradable cross-linked polyacrylamide hydrogel and is 97.5% water and 2.5% dry matter. It is injected using a urethroscope under direct vision.

The safety and efficacy of Bulkamid has now been reported in both European and North American trials. A two-year European study of 135 women has reported a subjective responder rate of 64%, which was compatible with the 67% responder rate at 12 months, and this was supported by a significant decrease in incontinence episodes, frequency, and urinary leakage. The overall reinjection rate was 35% and there were no long-term safety concerns.

These results are supported by a large prospective single-blind, randomised controlled study comparing Bulkamid to collagen in 229 North American women at 33 centres. At 12-month follow up, responder rates, defined as a greater than 50% reduction in leakage and incontinence episodes, were 53.2% in the Bulkamid arm and 55.4% in the collagen arm. Dry rates at 12 months were 47.5 and 50%, respectively.

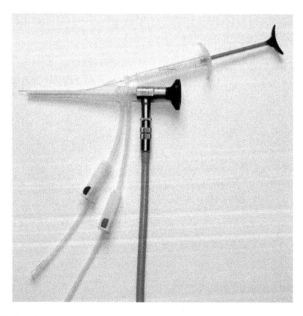

Figure 7.2 Bulkamid.

Coaptite

Coaptite (Boston Scientific) (Figure 7.3) is a particulate bulking agent composed of calcium hydroxylapatite particles and is injected using a cystoscopic technique. Coaptite has been compared to collagen in a 12-month prospective randomised comparative study of 231 women. At 12 months, 63.4% of the Coaptite group showed improvement of one Stamey grade or more compared to 57% in the Collagen group. In addition, re-injection rates were 62% in the Coaptite arm as compared to 73.9% in the collagen arm, and there were no long-term safety concerns.

Durasphere

Durasphere (Coloplast) (Figure 7.4) is a particulate bulking agent composed of pyrolytic carbon coated beads, which is injected using a trans-urethral or peri-urethral technique. Durasphere has been compared to collagen in a multicentre,

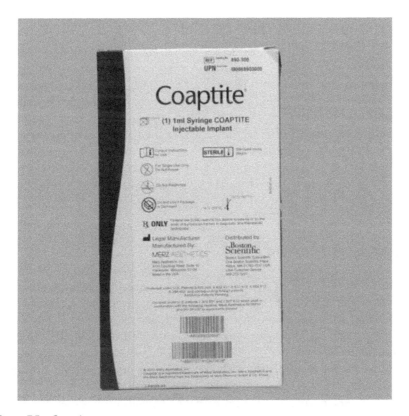

Figure 7.3 Coaptite.

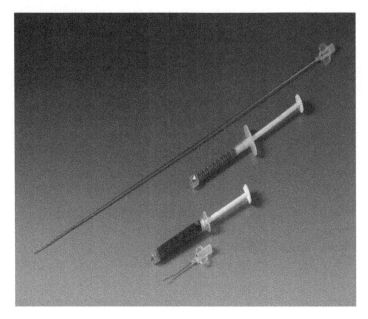

Figure 7.4 Durasphere.

randomised, double-blind controlled trial of 355 women with ISD. At 12 months, 80.3% of the Durasphere group reported improvement in Stamey grade or more compared to 69.1% in the collagen group. Although adverse effects were similar between groups, there were more cases of urgency and urinary retention reported in the Durasphere arm. Subsequently, 56 women from one centre were followed up over 36 months. Treatment was initially effective in 63% of women and this fell to 33% at 24 months and 21% at 36 months compared to 19% and 9% for collagen, respectively.

Urolastic

Urolastic (Urogyn) (Figure 7.5) is a homogeneous bulking agent composed of vinyl dimethyl terminated polydimethylsiloxane polymer, tetrapropoxysilane cross-linking agent, platinum vinyl tetramethyl siloxane complex catalyst and titanium dioxide radiopacifying agent and is injected peri-urethrally using an application device. In a small proof of concept study of 20 women, a dry rate of 68% was reported at 12 months with corresponding improvements in health-related quality of life (HRQoL) and pad weights. There was, however, a complication rate of 30% including pain and dyspareunia, and dry rates fell to 45% at

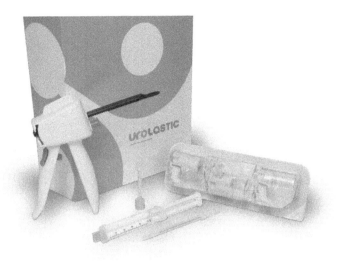

Figure 7.5   Urolastic.

24 months. A larger study of 105 women has also reported objective success rates of 59.3% and improvement rates of 71.4% at 12 months, although, here again success rates fell to 32.7% at 24 months with a complication rate of 25.8%.

More recently, a systematic review and meta-analysis of five papers has been performed, which reported an objective success rate of 32.7–67% with a mean of 57% and a subjective improvement in 80% of patients.

Urolon

Urolon (Aqlane Medical) (Figure 7.6) is a polycaprolactone based bio-resorbable urethral bulking agent that is thought to stimulate collagen production and is injected cystoscopically. The efficacy and safety of Urolon has been reported in a small multi-centre trial of 50 patients followed up over 12 months. Improvement using the Stamey Grading Score was recorded in 57.9% of patients at 12 months with a cure rate of 39.5%. There was a corresponding improvement in patient-related outcome and HRQoL with no reported significant adverse events.

Single Incision Mini-Slings (SIMS)

The description of the Integral Theory and subsequent introduction of retropubic and trans obturator mid-urethral slings has revolutionised continence surgery. More recently there has been a move to a minimally invasive approach in the

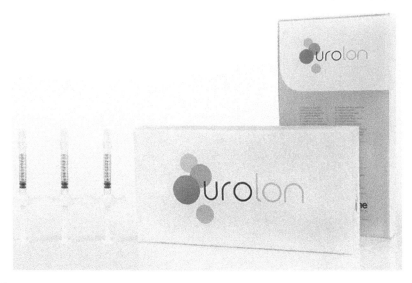

Figure 7.6 Urolon.

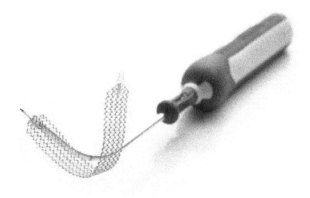

Figure 7.7 Solyx.

ambulatory setting using single incision mini-slings (SIMS), which are associated with a lower incidence of bladder perforation and may be performed under local anaesthesia. Although several SIMS were developed, many have now been withdrawn from the market. Solyx (Boston Scientific) (Figure 7.7), Ajust (Bard) (Figure 7.8) and Ophira (Promedon) (Figure 7.9) are still available in some countries.

A systematic review and meta-analysis comparing SIMS with standard midurethral slings reviewed 26 randomised controlled trials including 3308 women.

Figure 7.8 Ajust.

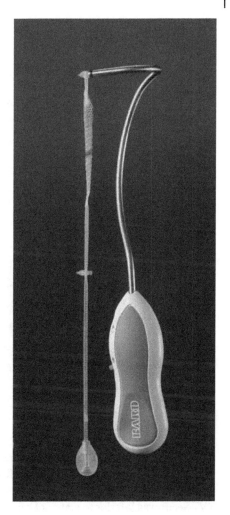

After excluding TVT Secur (now withdrawn), there was no significant difference in patient-reported cure (RR: 0.94; 95% CI: 0.88–1.00) and objective cure (RR: 0.98; 95% CI: 0.94–1.01) at a mean follow up of 18.6 months between the two procedures. Although SIMS were associated with less post-operative pain and an earlier return to normal activities, there was a trend to higher rates of repeat continence surgery (RR: 2.00; 95%CI: 0.93–4.31).

More recently, a further systematic review and meta-analysis has been reported by the Cochrane group and assessed 31 trials involving 3290 women including those trials assessing TVT Secur. Overall, women were more likely to remain incontinent after SIMS when compared to retropubic TVT slings (RR: 2.08; 95% CI: 1.04–4.14)

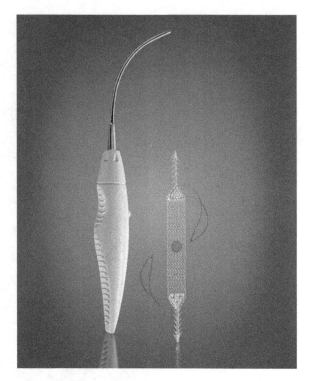

Figure 7.9   Ophira.

and trans obturator slings (RR: 2.55; 95% CI: 1.93–3.36). In addition, there was a higher risk of vaginal mesh exposure (RR: 3.75; 95% CI: 1.42–9.86) and bladder/urethral erosion (RR: 17.79; 95% CI: 1.06–298.88). The authors concluded that TVT Secur was inferior to standard mid-urethral slings and that there were insufficient data to allow reliable comparisons between the other SIMS and standard slings.

Synthetic Mid-urethral Slings

The use of synthetic slings, either as a retropubic approach (using TVT) or a transobturator approach (using TVT-O), had largely replaced the traditional incontinence procedures in the last two decades. The efficacy of it has been proven in many studies. Following the reports in the media on mesh-related complications in prolapse surgeries and the subsequent FDA warning, the general public has become fearful of the mid-urethral sling. In the UK, this has led to a temporary ban on the use of tension-free synthetic slings until more data becomes available. If, on further information, synthetic mid-urethral slings become the procedure of choice, its greatest advantage would be the possibility of doing an effective procedure in an ambulatory setting.

Thermomodulation

There is currently increasing interest in the use of thermo-modulation devices as ambulatory procedures for managing women with SUI. The evidence supporting the use of laser therapy and radiofrequency is, however, currently limited.

Laser

There are currently two different types of laser that are being used clinically within urogynaecology; Micro ablative fractional CO_2 laser (MonaLisa Touch, Deka) (Figure 7.10) and non-ablative photothermal Erbium: YAG laser (Er: YAG-laser) (Fotona Smooth, Fotona) (Figure 7.11). Both types of laser cause thermo-modulation by heating and, in the case of the CO_2 laser, ablating columns of tissue. This leads to a controlled temperature rise, which results in vasodilatation, collagen remodelling, collagen synthesis, neo-vascularisation and elastin formation. This improves vaginal elasticity and restoration of vaginal flora to premenopausal status.

Although there is increasing evidence to support the use of laser therapy in the management of women with genitourinary syndrome of menopause (GSM), there is a paucity of evidence supporting usage in patients with SUI. A small prospective randomised controlled trial comparing Er: YAG laser to sham therapy has recently been reported in 114 premenopausal women. At three-month follow-up there was a significant improvement in subjective outcome in the laser arm with dry rates of 21% as compared to 4% in the sham arm. A further small nonrandomised study has compared Er: YAG laser to TVT or TOT in 100 patients. Overall, there were comparable improvements in the 1-hour pad test and HRQoL, although the dry rates were significantly lower in the laser arm when compared to the TVT and TOT arm (50%, 69%, and 68%, respectively).

Consequently, whilst laser therapy may be considered as an ambulatory treatment for women with SUI, women need to be counselled regarding the lack of robust evidence and the need for ongoing long-term clinical trials.

Figure 7.10   Monalisa Touch Laser, Deka.

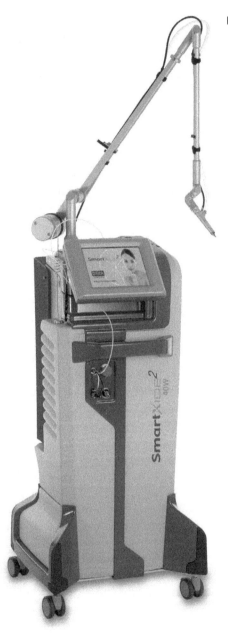

Figure 7.11 Fotona Smooth, Fotona.

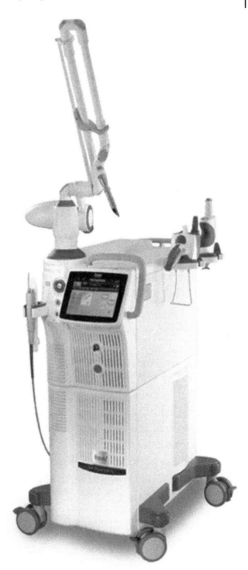

Radiofrequency

Radiofrequency devices emit focused electromagnetic waves that generate heat upon meeting tissue impedance. At tissue temperatures between 40–45 °C, radiofrequency can induce fibroblasts to produce collagen through activation of heat shock proteins and initiation of the inflammatory cascade. Ex-vivo and in-vivo studies have demonstrated that radiofrequency treatment produces thickening and rearrangement of collagen and elastin fibres with no reported adverse events in the epidermis, nerves, or blood vessels.

The safety and efficacy of radio frequency collagen denaturation has been assessed in a number of small retrospectives series. A three-year follow-up of 21 patients reported that 56% of patients achieved a 50% or greater reduction in incontinence episode frequency with no long-term adverse effects. These results are supported by a larger prospective study in 139 women which reported a subjective improvement in HRQoL, although, it did not evaluate outcome with any objective measures.

The Cochrane group has recently published a systematic review and meta-analysis of transurethral radiofrequency collagen denaturation in the management of women with SUI. Overall, only one sham controlled randomised trial of 173 women was suitable for analysis and, given the limitations of this study, the authors concluded that the role of radiofrequency collagen denaturation in the treatment of women with SUI remains unclear.

Conclusion

Minimally invasive therapies have revolutionised the surgical management of SUI and many may now be performed as ambulatory procedures under local anaesthesia. Ambulatory care minimises cost within the healthcare system, reduces morbidity, and improves the patient experience. This results in an earlier return to normal activities and hence an economic benefit to society beyond the healthcare system.

Although the role of urethral bulking agents is well established, the precise role of SIMS remains to be determined, and many devices have now been withdrawn from the market.

Newer therapies continue to be developed, and there may be a role for laser therapy and radiofrequency in the management of SUI. However, at present there is a paucity of evidence for these new modalities and there remains a need for robust clinical trials.

Further Reading

Blaivis, J.G. and Olsson, C.A. (1988). Stress incontinence: classification and surgical approach. *J. Urol.* 139: 727–731.

DeLancey, J.O. (1994). Structural support of the urethra as it relates to stress incontinence: the hammock hypothysis. *Am. J. Obstet. Gynaecol.* 170: 1713–1720.

Hannestad, Y.S., Rortveit, G., Sandvik, H., and Hunskar, S. (2000). A community-based epidemiological survey of female urinary incontinence: The Norwegian EPINCONT Study. *J. Clin. Epidemiol.* 53: 1150–1157.

Haylen, B.T., de Ridder, D., Freeman, R.M. et al. (2010). An International Urogynaecological Association (IUGA)/International Continence Society (ICS) joint report on the terminology for female pelvic floor dysfunction. *Int. Urogynecol. J.* 21: 5–26.

8

Pelvic Organ Prolapse Surgery as an Ambulatory Procedure

Marcella Zanzarini Sanson and G. Willy Davila

Urogynaecological procedures are particularly well served as ambulatory procedures because most can be done via the vaginal approach, the anaesthetic time and surgical duration are rather brief, and post-operative pain does not often limit discharge. In the United States, the Centers for Medicare and Medicaid Services (CMS – the national insurance plan for retirees) has classified most urogynecological procedures including vaginal hysterectomy and mid-urethral slings as day-surgery procedures. Most private insurance companies have followed suit and as a consequence, the standard of care in the United States is that most pelvic reconstructive procedures performed vaginally are performed as day-care procedures.

We have reported on our experience with a model of all vaginal procedures being performed as ambulatory same-day surgeries. Overall, clinical outcomes are not negatively impacted, although, patient acceptance and satisfaction are greatly dependent on pre-operative education.

Outside of the United States, institutions have followed this pattern of shifting pelvic floor surgeries to the outpatient setting. Similar positive results in terms of clinical outcomes and patient satisfaction have been reported.

This chapter will review the many steps pelvic reconstructive surgeons have taken, to safely and efficiently perform pelvic reconstructive surgeries as ambulatory day-surgery cases.

General Requirements

In ambulatory surgical procedures, general peri-operative considerations have to be followed. These include avoidance of medications with anti-coagulant properties, avoidance of pre-operative constipation, and the implementation of enhanced recovery after surgery protocols (ERAS). Addressing specific aspects in the

Ambulatory Urology and Urogynaecology, First Edition. Edited by Abhay Rane and Ajay Rane.
© 2021 John Wiley & Sons Ltd. Published 2021 by John Wiley & Sons Ltd.

urogynaecological procedures and adopting ERAS protocols can make prolapse surgeries amenable to ambulatory care. The patient and her family should be involved in the decision to perform a procedure in the ambulatory setting.

Enhanced Recovery Protocols

ERAS protocols utilise multidisciplinary teams to optimise patient outcomes with improved patient satisfaction and decreased hospital costs. ERAS protocols have been applied to urogynecologic surgery as well, with a positive impact being noted. Overall, when compared to traditional management, no significant differences were noted, except that ERAS patients were more likely to be discharged with a urinary catheter and had a slightly higher readmission rate but patient satisfaction was high.

The essentials of ERAS protocols are based on four stages, all aiming to reduce surgical stress, maintain normal physiological function perioperatively, and expedite post-operative recovery (see Table 8.1).

The First Stage for ERAS is Pre-admission

The pre-operative phase is an opportunity to educate patients, set expectations of what will occur before, during, and after the surgery. This includes a discussion regarding postoperative pain and a management strategy (see Table 8.2).

At the time, the patient is advised to reduce alcohol consumption and quit smoking. Smoking cessation four weeks before surgery has been associated with fewer peri- and post-operative complications.

All medications, medical conditions, and nutritional status should be optimised before surgery.

Precise ambulatory surgery protocols largely rely on the participation of the patient, her family, and the entire clinical team in order to achieve a successful and complication-free ambulatory procedure. Preoperative discharge planning is key to a successful ambulatory vaginal surgery programme. Supportive family or friends will make recovery much more pleasant for the patient and this should be explored in the pre-admission discussion. Frequently, family members include elderly spouses who may not be comfortable caring for a patient during the first few days after surgery. Education regarding pain-medication dosing, assistance with ambulation, presence of vaginal bleeding, among other details specific to the procedure should be discussed during the informed-consent process prior to surgery.

A significant proportion of patients following a urogynaecological surgery may go home with a urinary catheter, and the possibility of post-operative

Table 8.1 Enhanced recovery after surgery (ERAS) protocol stages.

Stage of ERAS	Area of Focus	Intervention/Meds
Pre-admission	Patient education Medical optimization Reduce alcohol consumption and stop smoking Nutritional and physical condition Explore home support	
Pre-operative	Reduce fasting time Avoid mechanical bowel preparation Analgesia	• 8 oz (250 ml) carbohydrate beverage 2–4 h before surgery. • No solids after midnight. Clear liquids diet 2–4 h before surgery. • Acetaminophen (paracetamol), NSAID, Gabapentin
Intra-operative	Minimally invasive surgery Non-opioid analgesia Euvolemia Normothermia PONV prophylaxis	• Local infiltration • Acetaminophen (paracetamol) • Ketamine • Scopolamine transdermal Patch/ Dexamethasone
Post-operative	Mobilisation Euvolemia Early dispositive removal Early oral intake Multimodal analgesia	• Acetaminophen (paracetamol) • NSAIDs • Oral opioids as needed

catheterization should be discussed. Up to 60% of patients undergoing pelvic floor surgery will need catheter drainage beyond the first day, so all should be made aware of the possibility of going home with a catheter. A frank discussion pre-operatively regarding this is the key to managing expectations and to avoid a disappointed or unhappy patient.

The Second Stage of ERAS is Pre-operative

Preoperative fasting increases catabolism that may affect peri-operative outcomes. Reducing fasting to six hours for solid food and two hours for clear liquids improves surgical outcomes with no increased risk of aspiration. Pre-operative bowel preparation should be avoided for patients undergoing benign gynecologic procedures. Even though patients can experience a high level of anxiety before surgery, long-acting anxiolytics should be avoided. To minimise opioid exposure

Table 8.2 Peri-operative pain-management options.

Stage of ERAS	Medication options
Pre-operative treatment	Celecoxib 400 mg PO Gabapentin 600 mg PO
PONV prophylaxis	Dexamethasone 4–8 mg IV at incision Ondansetron 4 mg before incision closure
Intra-operative analgesia	Per anaesthesia routine IV acetaminophen (paracetamol) IV Toradol Local lidocaine Local bupivacaine liposome
Immediate post-operative pain	IV acetaminophen (paracetamol) 1 g every 6 h Celecoxib 200 mg PO every 12 h Gabapentin 300 mg PO every 8 h Toradol 15–30 mg iv every 6 h prn Hydromorphone 0.5–1.5 mg IV every 3 h prn
POD 1	After discontinuation of IV medication • Celecoxib 200 mg PO every 12 h • Gabapentin 300 mg PO every 8 h • Acetaminophen (paracetamol) 1 g PO every 6 h scheduled x 3 days (total) • Oxycodone 5–15 mg PO every 3 prn
Discharge	• Acetaminophen (paracetamol) 1 g PO every 6 h scheduled x 3 days (total) • Ibuprofen 600 mg PO every 6 h scheduled × 3 days as needed. • Oxycodone 5–15 mg PO every 4–6 h prn • Tramadol or Tapentadol 50 mg every 6 h

and control pain, multimodal non-opioid analgesia can be administered immediately before entering the operating room: Acetaminophen (paracetamol, 1000 mg PO), Gabapentin (600–1200 mg PO) or Pregabalin (100–300 mg PO) and Celecoxib (200–400 mg PO) are examples of pre-emptive pain therapy.

The Third Stage of ERAS is Intra-operative

The anaesthetic protocol should allow for rapid recovery, including the use of short-acting anaesthetic agents or using regional anaesthesia where possible. Most vaginal procedures do not require paralysis or intubation. If performed in an ambulatory surgical centre, where prompt room turnover and patient traffic is a requirement, intravenous sedation with a laryngeal mask airway (LMA) may be appropriate, along with local anaesthetic infiltration of the surgical field. In POP surgeries, a spinal block containing bupivacaine plus hydromorphone (50–100 µg) or a light general anaesthetic with intravenous sedation will normally suffice. Regional anaesthesia (spinal/epidural) is suitable for most pelvic procedures, but the time it takes for the block to wear off may negatively impact on patient flow and can increase the likelihood of discharge with a urinary catheter.

In vaginal surgery, the intra-operative use of Allen-type supportive stirrups reduces the likelihood of neurologic complications and optimises the surgeon's access to the pelvis.

Preventing intra-operative hypothermia helps keep blood pressure stable during surgery. Normothermia prevents a delay in wound healing and decreases the risk of surgical infection, blood loss, and cardiac morbidity. ERAS protocols emphasise the concept of euvolemia, as fluid overload contributes to peripheral and visceral edema and electrolyte abnormalities. Hypovolemia, affecting cardiac output and tissue oxygenation, should be avoided.

Intra-operative analgesia is important for appropriate post-operative pain management. A small dose of Ketamine (0.5 mg/kg bolus at induction and closure, and an infusion of 10 µg/kg/min) was shown to reduce pain score and opioid use in the post-operative phase. Local anaesthetics (i.e., 1% lidocaine with epinephrine) used at the incision site can reduce acute post-operative pain, however, the short duration of actions may limit the benefits. An intravenous dose of Ketorolac (Toradol) prior to transfer to the recovery room reduces the need for opioids.

Intravenous dexamethasone (4–8 mg) should be considered as prophylaxis for post-operative nausea and vomiting (PONV). Managing nausea and vomiting enhances the early recovery by improving subjective mood. Anecdotal reports that dexamethasone is safe and useful peri-operatively has been tested via randomised trials, and many ERAS protocols now implement this medication.

Urinary retention is one of the barriers to performing urogynaecological procedures as day-care surgery. Apart from pre-operative counselling, alternatives to transurethral catheter drainage can be considered. This can include pre-operative education on intermittent self-catheterization or the intra-operative placement of a suprapubic catheter. Currently, there are no clear pre-operative predictors for identifying which patient may require prolonged post-operative catheter drainage. Recognised risk factors include pre-operative urinary retention, abnormal pressure voiding studies and uroflowmetry, performance of posterior colporrhaphy, and tensioned pubo-vaginal sling.

The Fourth Stage of ERAS is Post-operative

Post-operative interventions aim to reduce patient discomfort and expedite recovery. Early mobilisation is a key component of all post-operative-care protocols. It improves pulmonary and bowel function, and decreases muscle wasting. The removal of movement-limiting devices such as catheters, drains, and IV tubing as soon as possible is directly related to facilitating mobility and pain control. A progressive increase in oral intake reduces the requirement for intravenous hydration and decreases the risk of post-operative ileus.

Pain management is essential in ERAS and day-care procedures. Most post-operative pain can be at least partially managed with non-opioid medications. Acetaminophen and NSAIDs can reduce opioid consumption without compromising pain control. These medications in conjunction with pre-operative corticosteroids should be considered. Once needed, oral opioid administration is preferred to parenteral. Even though opioids are potent pain relievers that can be used for post-operative pain, narcotics commonly have predictable side effects including nausea, vomiting, and constipation. They can also induce dependency and addiction.

PONV causes patient discomfort and a prolonged hospital stay. For this reason, ERAS protocols should include not only nausea and vomiting prophylaxis but also a clear treatment plan for when it occurs post-operatively. The application of a trans-dermal scopolamine patch, alone or in combination with other medications, is effective for PONV control.

Some ambulatory care centres are equipped with a post-recovery room. A post-recovery room (phase II) is an observation area where patients can be transferred for a period of additional monitoring or care before deciding if same day discharge is appropriate. This additional period of monitoring allows the effects of a spinal anaesthetic to wear off, time to ensure a patient is safely mobilising, treatment of ongoing nausea or vomiting, and provision of additional pain relief. It is also a suitable setting to ensure a patient is adequately voiding, and replace a catheter or teach intermittent self-catheterisation if necessary. Any barriers to home discharge can be identified and addressed in phase II. If a longer period of care is required, the patient can be either admitted or transferred to another care facility depending on the capabilities of the particular surgical practice.

Urogynaecological Procedures

Most urogynaecological procedures that are approached vaginally can be performed as day surgery procedures. However, individual variables such as chronic pulmonary disease, impaired mobility, cognitive dysfunction, and significant cardiac disease may not be appropriate for ambulatory care.

Vaginal Hysterectomy

Vaginal hysterectomy is commonly performed as surgical management of pelvic organ prolapse. Until recently, it was not considered a day-surgery procedure; however, with the need to reduce surgical wait times, the thinking and practice has changed. Although a major surgical procedure, the need for prolonged hospitalisation has been challenged with the advent of evidence-based protocols ensuring patient safety when performed in the outpatient setting. After a vaginal hysterectomy, the indwelling catheter is often left in place. The post-operative use of an indwelling catheter after vaginal hysterectomy is a routine practice citing close proximity of the operative field to bladder. This routine practice has been challenged by studies showing that indwelling catheterization after vaginal hysterectomy is not necessary.

Adopting the vaginal hysterectomy as a day-care procedure has not shown an increased complication rate, even when the adnexa is removed vaginally. Ensuring haemostasis of all pedicles and appropriate closure of the vaginal cuff forms the mainstay of intra-operative safety. The use of electrosurgical bipolar vessel sealing in vaginal hysterectomy has shown to reduce the operative time, intra-operative blood loss, and post-operative pain which also facilitates day-care surgery.

Utilising laparoscopy to assist in vaginal hysterectomy (Vaginal Natural Orifice TransEndoscopic Surgery – vNOTES) can further increase the success in performing it as an ambulatory procedure. Protocols have been published in the hope of optimising outcomes for outpatient hysterectomy.

Anterior and Posterior Vaginal Repair (Colporrhaphy)

Performing vaginal repairs as day-case procedures was proposed as early as 1995 by J.R. Miklos. Native tissue repairs with dissection and plication of the pubocervical and recto-vaginal fascia in anterior and posterior colporraphy, respectively, are the most amenable to ambulatory repair. To start with, both these procedures can be performed using local anaesthesia. Hydro-dissection using Bupivacaine 0.25% with 1 : 200 000 adrenaline, helps assist fascial dissection and effective haemostasis. In an anterior repair, the simple plication of fascia ensures that post-operative pain is easily managed with simple non-opioid analgesics.

Posterior colporrhaphy or posterior repair entails not only restoration of anterior rectal support but also normalisation of the vaginal introitus calibre. It is this part of the procedure that can pose a challenge when performed in an ambulatory setting. In order to normalise vaginal calibre, the laterally displaced endopelvic fascia, perineal muscle, and occasionally pelvic floor musculature must be plicated in the midline. This plication can lead to posterior vaginal and perineal pain secondary to levator spasm and hyper tonus. Pain control can be obtained in the short term with intra-operative injection of a long-lasting local anaesthetic such as bupivacaine, although, not all studies have demonstrated a significant benefit. Frequently, spasms of the levator musculature require opioid analgesia and additional smooth/striated muscle relaxants such as cyclobenzaprine.

The risk of major complications after vaginal repair is reported to be very low. A study of the efficacy of repairs done under local anaesthesia has shown that there is 63–80% improvement on POP-Q scores.

Vault Suspension Procedures

Vault suspension procedures can be performed via the abdominal or vaginal route, with the abdominal route posing more challenges in the ambulatory setting. Sacrospinous ligament fixation (SSLF) is a safe and effective technique for vaginal support. Pre-operative bowel preparation, adequate dissection of the para-rectal space, exposure of the sacrospinous ligament and proper suture positioning are essential components in SSLF. The procedure can be associated with temporary buttock pain and consideration can be given to injection of local anaesthetic into the ligaments. Intraperitoneal uterosacral ligament suspension requires entrance into the peritoneal cavity and packing of the bowel contents. As such, this may require deeper anaesthesia during the procedure to manage greater discomfort from peritoneal irritation. Nevertheless, patient satisfaction is high with this method of vault suspension as an ambulatory procedure.

Abdominal sacro-colpopexy, the gold standard for vaginal vault suspension, requires prolonged general anaesthesia, abdominal incisions, bowel preparations and packing, and mesh anchorage, all of which may not be suitable for the ambulatory setting. Recently, the feasibility of laparoscopic or robotic sacro-colpopexy as day-care surgery has been analysed and protocols have been developed and validated. The required general anaesthesia, deep Trendelenburg positioning and prolonged surgical time may, however, impact the practicality and safety of these procedures when performed as ambulatory procedures.

There are circumstances under which an open abdominal procedure can be accomplished as a day-surgery procedure. Appropriate patient selection, pre-operative counselling, an ERAS protocol, pre-incision local anaesthetic infiltration, and wound infiltration with bupivacaine liposome or usage of an ON-Q pump (elastomeric local anaesthetic pump) allows for sufficient pain control for same-day discharge. In general, most will use a 23-hour stay option to keep these patients overnight.

Obliterative Colpocleisis

Prolapse in the advanced elderly with medical co-morbidities pose surgical challenges. A LeFort-type colpocleisis performed under spinal or light general anaesthesia has been shown to be extremely safe and effective in this patient population. This procedure can have marked benefits on a patient's quality of life through improvement in urinary retention, vaginal ulceration, and recurrent urinary tract infections. A case series of women undergoing a colpocleisis, with the majority being done as day-surgery procedures, showed minimal morbidity and extremely high success rates.

Fistulae

Most vesical-vaginal and recto-vaginal fistulae in developed countries are small and amenable to ambulatory management. When counselled appropriately, the need for post-operative catheterisation is not a barrier. Complex fistulae and those in regions where access to medical care is limited, or when social barriers to care are present it should not be undertaken in the ambulatory care setting.

Practical Considerations to Grow an Ambulatory Urogynaecological Surgery Practice

Most vaginal and laparoscopic urogynaecological procedures are amenable to ambulatory surgical management. Protocols need to be adopted and followed by the entire care-provider team in order to be safe and effective. Patients need to be educated and counselled pre-operatively regarding the implications of ambulatory surgery, focusing on the importance of home-care providers, pain control, and possible need for discharge home with a urinary catheter in place. There needs to be appropriate follow-up care for all patients and in particular those that need to be discharged with a catheter in-situ.

For day-case vaginal repair surgery to be successful, it should be safe, acceptable, and preferable to patients. There must be adequate protocols in place for bladder care, out-of-hours access for advice, and admission to the gynaecology ward in case of any problems requiring overnight stay. Once same-day discharge programmes are implemented for urogynecologic procedures, outcomes and safety measures have to be audited regularly including patient acceptance and satisfaction.

Further Reading

(2018). ACOG Committee Opinion No. 750 summary: perioperative pathways: enhanced recovery after surgery. *Obstet. Gynecol.* 132 (3): 801–802.

Alas, A., Espaillat-Rijo, L.M., Plowright, L. et al. (2016). Same-day surgery for pelvic organ prolapse and urinary incontinence: assessing patient satisfaction and morbidity. *Perioper. Care Oper. Room Manag.* 5: 20–26.

Alas, A., Hidalgo, R., Espaillat, L. et al. (2019). Does spinal anesthesia lead to postoperative urinary retention in same-day urogynecologic surgery? A retrospective review. *Int Urogynecol J* 30: 1283–1289.

Carey, E.T. and Moulder, J.K. (2018). Perioperative management and implementation of enhanced recovery programs in gynecologic surgery for benign indications. *Obstet. Gynecol.* 132: 137–146.

Ghoshal, S. and Smith, A.R. (2005). Ambulatory surgery in urogynecology. *Best Pract. Res. Clin. Obstet. Gynecol.* 19: 769–777.

Miklos, J.R., Sze, E.H.M., and Karram, M.M. (1995). Vaginal correction of pelvic organ relaxation using local anesthesia. *Obstet Gynecol* 86 (6): 922–924.

Papa Petros, P.E. (1998). Development of generic models for ambulatory vaginal surgery – a preliminary report. *Int. Urogynecol. J. Pelvic Floor Dysfunct.* 9: 19–27.

Rodriguez Trowbridge, E., Evans, S.L., Sarosiek, B.M. et al. (2019). Enhanced recovery program for minimally invasive and vaginal urogynecologic surgery. *Int. Urogynecol. J.* 30: 313–321.

Zebede, S., Smith, A.L., Plowright, L. et al. (2013). Obliterative LeFort Colpocleisis in a large group of elderly women. (incl. video). *Obstet Gynecol* 121: 279–284.

9

Common Urethral and Vaginal Lesions in Ambulatory Urogynaecology

Mugdha Kulkarni and Anna Rosamilia

Introduction

Benign urethral and vaginal lesions are commonly encountered in the urogynae-cology clinic setting. With the advent of ambulatory urogynaecology many of these conditions can be managed as day care procedures. This chapter will cover some of the common benign urethral and vaginal lesions: urethral caruncle, ure-thral prolapse, urethral diverticulum, urethral fistula, Skene's duct cyst, Bartholin's cyst, Gartner's duct cyst, and periurethral lesions. It is beyond the scope of this chapter to cover any malignant lesions.

A review of the embryology and anatomy of the urethra and vagina helps to understand the pathology and management of urethral and vaginal lesions.

Embryology and Anatomy of Urethra

The caudal portion of the vesicourethral canal forms the female urethra. It is 3–5 cm long and about 5–7 mm in diameter. The urethra is embedded in the adventitia of the anterior vaginal wall, perforates the perineal membrane and ends with the external orifice in the vestibule above the vaginal opening. The urethra has intrinsic and extrinsic sphincter mechanisms which aid in main-taining continence. Urethral smooth muscles, along with the detrusor from the bladder base form the intrinsic sphincter. The extrinsic sphincter is composed of two portions: the inner portion of striated muscles within and adjacent to the urethral wall and the outer portion of skeletal muscle fibres of the pelvic diaphragm.

Ambulatory Urology and Urogynaecology, First Edition. Edited by Abhay Rane and Ajay Rane.
© 2021 John Wiley & Sons Ltd. Published 2021 by John Wiley & Sons Ltd.

The urethra is surrounded by multiple periurethral ducts and glands. Skene's glands are adjacent to the distal urethra and are the largest. The urethra lies in close proximity to the vagina. Vaginal epithelium is lined by loose connective tissue called lamina propria and does not contain any glands. Vaginal lubrication occurs as a transudate from vessels, cervix, and the Bartholin's and Skene's glands.

Benign Urethral Lesions

Urethral Caruncle

A urethral caruncle is the most common female urethral lesion and is usually seen in post-menopausal women. It is a benign condition resulting from the eversion of the distal portion of the posterior urethral meatus. A caruncle is usually small, soft, smooth or friable, and bright pink to dark. Usually single, it can be pedunculated and grow up to 1–2 cm long. Histologically, a caruncle contains blood vessels, loose connective tissue and is covered by urothelium and squamous epithelium. The pathogenesis of a urethral caruncle is not clearly understood. It is thought to result from oestrogen deficiency in the postmenopausal woman leading to atrophy of urothelium and retraction of the vagina.

Most women are asymptomatic and caruncles are usually an incidental finding on genital examination. Though most often seen in postmenopausal women, it can also occur in premenopausal and prepubertal girls. Symptoms described have been that of a lump, bleeding, dysuria, and pain.

A study looked at the effects of asymptomatic caruncles on micturition and found that 6%of women who presented with urinary incontinence were noted to have caruncles, but there was no effect on micturition when caruncles measured<1 cm. However, some sources have reported voiding dysfunction in association with a caruncle.

Diagnosis is clinical and based on the characteristic appearance of a pink, soft, sessile or pedunculated mass protruding from the urethral meatus, usually on the posterior aspect. Biopsy is not necessary unless diagnosis is uncertain or if there is a suspicion of malignancy.

There are no large studies or randomised controlled trials (RCTs) evaluating various treatment strategies. Asymptomatic women do not require treatment. A conservative approach with regular clinical observation or self-observation is suggested. In women who are symptomatic, initial management is topical oestrogen cream for two to three months. In cases of large, persistent lesions, speciality referral to a urogynaecologist or urologist should be considered. If initial therapy of topical oestrogen fails, surgical treatment can be offered. Surgical treatment involves initial cystourethroscopy to assess the urethra and bladder, followed by catheterisation. Removal of a caruncle is either by excision and ligation or diathermy of the base under local or general anaesthesia. Following the procedure, the patient can be discharged home with an indwelling catheter for planned removal in the next 24–48 hours. Risks associated with the procedure include bleeding or rarely external urethral meatal stenosis.

Urethral Prolapse

Urethral prolapse is uncommon and defined as eversion of the urethral mucosa circumferentially through the distal urethra. It is usually seen in prepubertal and postmenopausal women. One theory suggests that prolapse occurs as a result of separation of the two muscular layers of the urethra, which can be congenital or acquired. Other theories are similar to the one proposed for urethral caruncle, based on a lack of oestrogen leading to urothelium atrophy and retraction of the vaginal epithelium. This also fits with the bimodal age distribution. Urethral prolapse can also occur as a consequence of obstetric trauma.

Prepubertal girls are usually asymptomatic and this is an incidental finding on examination. The most common symptom is vaginal bleeding along with a urethral mass. In contrast, postmenopausal women are often symptomatic with vaginal bleeding and voiding symptoms being a common presentation.

Diagnosis is by clinical examination. The urethral prolapse appears as a circumferential, small doughnut shaped mass protruding from the anterior vaginal wall with the external urethral meatus in the middle (Figure 9.1). It can be erythematous, congested, infected, or even ulcerated.

Postmenopausal women are usually treated initially with topical oestrogen therapy, but if unresponsive or large, surgical excision should be considered. Excisional biopsy should be considered and is mandatory if malignancy is suspected. Surgical excision is indicated for young symptomatic patients and for recurrent urethral prolapse.

An indwelling Foley catheter at the beginning of the procedure is helpful, though it may be difficult to place it when tissue is oedematous. The prolapsed mucosal tissue is excised using scissors or cautery in a circumferential manner. Using stay sutures around the mucosa at 12, 3, and 9 o'clock position during the excision helps in traction and prevents the mucosal edge from retracting. The urethral mucosa and the vaginal tissue edges are approximated with interrupted sutures as the excision proceeds from anterior to posterior with 4–0 vicryl. The catheter is left in place for 24 hours but patients can be discharged home the same day, with adequate analgesia.

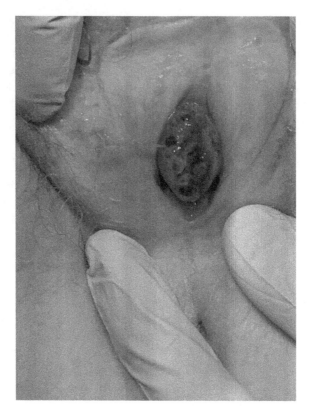

Figure 9.1 Urethral prolapse.

Urethral Diverticulum

A urethral diverticulum is the localised outpouching of the urethral mucosa into the surrounding non-urothelial tissues (Figure 9.2). This is a relatively uncommon condition and it is difficult to estimate its true prevalence due to the difficulty in diagnosis. Prevalence reported on basis of a urethrography series is 1–5%.

Urethral diverticula can be congenital or acquired. The congenital diverticulae are thought to be remnants of the Gartner's duct, but most are likely to be acquired rather than congenital. The proposed theory is that the diverticulum develops as a result of chronic infection of periurethral glands. This subsequently leads to obstruction and enlargement of glands and abscess formation. Once this abscess ruptures into the urethral lumen, it leads to a communication between the two forming a diverticulum. Various studies have supported this theory, finding chronic inflammation on histology that results

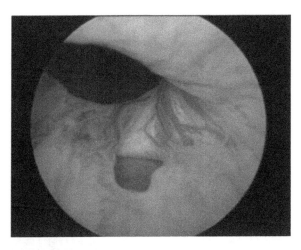

Figure 9.2 Urethral diverticulum on cystoscopy.

in fibrosis within and surrounding the diverticulum. Other theories proposed are trauma or injury during childbirth or vaginal and urethral surgery. A diverticular opening into the urethra from a small diverticulum is usually via a single ostium but it is not unusual to find multiple ostia and loculated diverticulae.

The symptoms are highly variable. The most common symptoms are lower urinary tract complaints of frequency and urgency, in addition to recurrent urinary tract infections and dysuria. The classic triad of dyspareunia, post-micturition dribble, and dysuria are seen in approximately 35% of patients. Haematuria, urinary incontinence, vaginal mass, vaginal pain, discharge, and urinary retention can be other symptoms of an urethral diverticulum.

Diagnosis requires a high index of suspicion. Apart from history, a thorough physical examination is essential because, in most cases, there will be a palpable mass in the sub-urethral region in the anterior vaginal wall. Diverticulae are usually present in the distal or middle portion of the posterior aspect of the urethra, about 2–3 cm proximal to the urethral opening. The pathognomonic finding of urethral discharge expressed by pressure on the suburethral mass is present in only 25% of cases. The mass is usually soft but can be firm to hard in the presence of a calculus or malignant change.

Investigations are helpful in differentiating a urethral diverticulum from other lesions such as vaginal wall cysts, cystocele, Skene's gland abnormalities, ectopic ureterocoele, vaginal leiomyomas and endometriosis. Urethroscopy with a 0- or 15° telescope and the urethrotome (Sachse) sheath can be valuable in identifying the ostia, but it is important to understand that in the presence of inflammatory changes, ostia may not be clearly visualised (Figure 9.3).

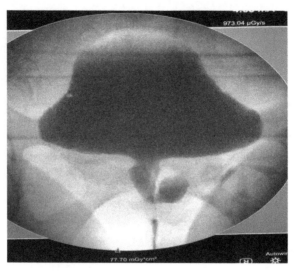

Figure 9.3 Diverticulum on cystogram.

Imaging in the form of a positive pressure urethrogram using a double balloon catheter forcing contrast into the diverticulae was the diagnostic technique of choice. Magnetic resonance imaging (MRI) currently seems to have the best diagnostic performance and helps to exclude other periurethral lesions. In the presence of resource implications, a transvaginal ultrasound (TV USG) has been found to be helpful. It is important to remember not to compress the urethra with the transvaginal probe. Translabial ultrasound is also a cost-effective imaging modality for identification of urethral diverticulum.

Management

Conservative treatment can be considered for women without bothersome symptoms. These include digital compression with application of pressure on the suburethral mass after voiding or periodic needle aspiration. In patients with recurrent UTIs, antibiotic prophylaxis is recommended. These might offer symptomatic relief; however, the anatomical defect will persist. Long-term outcomes for conservative treatment are not known.

Surgical treatment should be offered to women with persistent symptoms and in the presence of diverticulum complications such as calculi. Surgical options include urethral diverticulectomy, marsupialisation of the diverticular sac and transurethral widening of the ostia.

The potential complication of urethrovaginal fistula in these procedures decrees that adherence to good surgical principles, accurate reconstruction, and the operation being performed only by surgeons trained in these procedures can reduce the risk. A detailed pre-operative evaluation is essential and includes ruling out urinary tract infection and diverticular abscess at the time of the surgery. Accurate assessment regarding the size and number of diverticula, number of ostia and position of the ostia in relation to the urethra and bladder neck are important. Complex diverticulae such as multiple, large, loculated or saddle-shaped require extensive dissection and possibly the need in some units, to be combined with a fascial sling procedure. These may not be suitable for an ambulatory setting, but in experienced hands, a straight forward diverticulum with a single ostium is appropriate for a transvaginal diverticulectomy as a day care procedure. The need for bladder drainage is still relevant regardless of diverticulum size.

Transvaginal Diverticulectomy

Urethroscopy to identify the ostia in the urethra is followed by placement of a urethral catheter. A vertical or inverted U-shaped incision is made in the anterior vaginal wall over the diverticular swelling. The vaginal epithelium is mobilised and the underlying periurethral fascia is identified. The fascia is then incised separately and mobilised to create flaps on either side. The diverticular sac is then excised and a probe is passed to identify the ostia at the base of the diverticulum. The urethral defect is closed either transversely or vertically ensuring extra mucosal closure. This is followed by closure of the periurethral fascia in layers ('vest-over-pants' closure) with absorbable sutures.

The layered closure avoids overlying suture lines, thereby, reducing the tension in the repair. Occasionally a vascularised Martius or labial fat pad graft is placed over the fascial closure to augment the repair. Finally, the vaginal wall incision is approximated with absorbable suture. The patient can be sent home with either a suprapubic or transurethral catheter for 10–14 days. In women with pre-operative stress urinary incontinence evaluated with urodynamics, a fascial sling can be placed although some studies suggest a staged approach since in many cases, symptoms are resolved with diverticulum repair (Stav 2008). Synthetic slings are contraindicated due to the risk of erosion and fistula formation. Following a diverticulectomy, a success rate of up to 70% is quoted. The complications include recurrence, stress incontinence, urethral stricture, and urethrovaginal fistula.

Marsupialisation of Diverticulum

Marsupialisation of the urethral diverticular sac, also referred to as the Spence procedure, is recommended only in distal urethral diverticulum. The procedure involves the creation of a permanent opening of the diverticular sac into the vagina. An incision is made through the posterior wall of the urethra down to the diverticulum and through the anterior vaginal wall. This incision thus extends from the urethral orifice to the proximal extent of the diverticulum. The urethra and diverticulum are opened and a 4-0 absorbable suture is used to marsupialise the vaginal wall with urethral mucosa. The diverticulum sac is sutured onto the anterior vaginal wall. The cavity created can be packed to promote fibrosis. It is a simple procedure and technically a generous meatotomy amenable to an ambulatory setting. Complications include splayed stream and urethrovaginal fistula.

Transurethral Saucerisation of Diverticulum

This procedure is again confined to only distal single diverticulum. It involves endoscopic transurethral incision of the ostia at the floor of the urethra, converting the small neck into a wide opening. This allows the diverticulum to drain freely. Performing this procedure in mid or proximal urethra can compromise the continence mechanism. In women presenting with any sub-urethral swelling, it is important to rule out urethral diverticulum, a condition with both diagnostic and management challenges.

Urethral Fistula

Urogenital fistula is an abnormal communication between the female genital tract and the bladder, urethra, or ureters. Obstetric trauma is the leading cause of urogenital fistula in the developing world, whereas gynaecologic surgery (such as hysterectomy, carcinoma, or pelvic radiation) is responsible for most vesicovaginal or ureterovaginal fistulas in developed countries. Types of fistula depend on the anatomic location, with vesicovaginal fistula being three times more common than other types.

In this chapter, we will only focus on the urethral fistula, also referred to as the urethrovaginal fistula –an abnormal communication between the vagina and urethra.

Pathogenesis

In the developed world, urethrovaginal fistulas are encountered after attempted repair of urethral diverticulum, following anterior colporrhaphy or mid-urethral sling procedures, and after obstetric trauma following the use of rotational forceps. Less commonly, they can be congenital or caused by prolonged indwelling transurethral catheterisation. Although an acute urethrovaginal fistula can be caused by direct injury during trauma or secondary to dissection, clamp, or crush injury, delayed fistula formation can result from suture impingement, radiation, or a malignant process. The blood supply is compromised leading to necrosis and eventually tissue breakdown. This process may

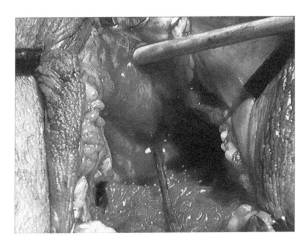

Figure 9.4   Urethrovaginal fistula.

progress over days to months before presentation. Very rarely, mid-urethral surgery may result in urethral erosion. Either the erosion itself or corrective surgery can lead to fistula formation.

Clinical features: Most women will present with painless urinary leakage. It can be intermittent but more often presents with continuous leakage with spraying of urine during voiding in some cases. The diagnosis is clinical and involves visualising urine leakage from the distal anterior 3–4 cm of the vagina. MRI may be considered for diagnosis of a complex urethral fistula. Cystourethroscopy, as a day procedure, helps in locating the fistulous opening and surgical planning (Figure 9.4).

Classification of Fistula

Summary of classification as standardised by Judith Goh and Kees Waaldijk:

Goh's classification is based on three variables –the length of the urethra (types 1–4), the size of the fistula (a–c) and the degree of scarring (I–III).

Urethral Length

Type 1	Distal edge of fistula >3.5 cm from the external urethral orifice (i.e., the urethra is not involved)
Type 2	Distal edge 2.5–3.5 cm from the external urethral orifice
Type 3	Distal edge 1.5–<2.5 cm from the external urethral orifice
Type 4	Distal edge <1.5 cm from the external urethral orifice

Fistula Size

(a)   <1.5 cm

(b)   1.5–3 cm

(c)   >3 cm

Scarring

Scarring I	No or mild fibrosis around fistula/vagina, and/or vagina length>6 cm or normal capacity
Scarring II	Moderate or severe fibrosis around fistula and/or vagina, and/or reduced vaginal length and/or capacity
Scarring III	Special considerations, e.g., circumferential fistula, previous repair

Treatment: Referral to a specialist with experience in fistula management is necessary. A small fistula diagnosed early can be managed conservatively with continuous bladder drainage that may assist in closure of the fistula. In most cases, however, surgical closure is indicated, and it is not usually amenable to an ambulatory procedure.

The surgical principles of urethrovaginal fistula closure are a tension-free closure repaired in layers. In a simple urethrovaginal fistula, after placing the transurethral catheter, a vaginal incision is made lateral to the fistulous opening, and the vaginal epithelium is mobilised. Using a 3-0 polyglactin suture, the urethral opening is approximated transversely with interrupted sutures in an extra mucosal fashion. Periurethral and then pubo-cervical fascia are then approximated, over the defect closure, to provide support, and finally the vaginal epithelium is closed. A Martius or labial fat pad or other graft may be considered if the fistula is large, recurrent, or complex. Post-operatively prolonged catheter drainage is needed.

Vaginal Lesions

Bartholin's Cyst

Bartholin's glands originate from the urogenital sinus. Obstruction of a Bartholin's duct is a prerequisite for cyst or abscess formation. This can occur as a consequence of infection or blockage from mucus. The cyst can be asymptomatic or present as a vaginal lump. In the presence of an infection, there is pain or dyspareunia.

The diagnosis is usually clinical. Bartholin's cysts are usually unilateral, 1–4 cm in diameter and located lateral to the introitus at 5 or 7 o'clock position medial to the labia minora. These lesions are easily visible on ultrasound, CT scan, or MRI; however, this is not necessary for diagnosis (Figure 9.5).

Management

Asymptomatic cysts can be offered conservative management. Symptomatic cysts or abscesses require surgical management under antibiotic cover. Marsupialization under anaesthesia is the preferred treatment to prevent reformation and maintain function. A vertical elliptical incision is made in the vestibular area close to the hymen allowing an oval edge of the vulval skin and cyst wall to be removed. The contents are drained and the cyst wall is sutured to the adjacent vulval skin using 3-0 absorbable sutures. The recurrence rate is around 10%.

An alternative technique is fistulisation using a Word catheter. A Word catheter is a 5.5 cm long, 15 Fr silicone catheter with a 3 cc balloon. The catheter is placed in the cyst or abscess through a 5 mm incision under local anaesthesia to aid drainage and epithelialization of the tract. The catheter is left in place for two to four weeks to allow drainage.

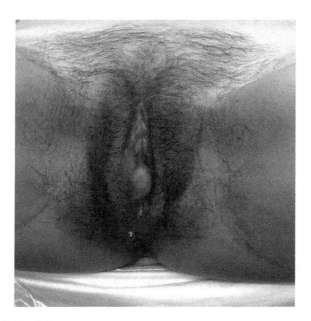

Figure 9.5 Bartholin's cyst.

The major complication of Bartholin's cyst is the risk of recurrence. In cases of repeated abscess or persistent cysts, removal of the Bartholin's gland can be recommended.

Gartner's and Müllerian Duct Cysts

The internal urogenital tract is derived from the Wolffian ducts (mesonephric) and the Müllerian ducts (paramesonephric). In women, during the eighth week of embryologic development, the paired Müllerian (paramesonephric) ducts fuse distally and develop into the uterus, cervix, and upper vagina. In addition, the Wolffian ducts regress. If the ducts persist in a vestigial form, they can form Gartner's cysts.

Gartner's duct cysts account for 11% of all vaginal cysts. These cysts are mainly located in the right anterolateral wall of the proximal third of the vagina. The Wolffian duct abnormality can also result in urinary tract abnormalities, such as ectopic ureter, unilateral renal dysgenesis, and renal hypoplasia.

Symptoms: Most are asymptomatic and are an incidental finding on examination, but they can enlarge in size and present as a vaginal lump and can be mistaken for pelvic organ prolapse. Other symptoms described are: dyspareunia, pain, vaginal discharge, or urinary symptoms due to extrinsic compression. Diagnosis is by clinical history and physical examination.

Histologically, a Gartner's cyst is lined by cuboidal low columnar, non-ciliated and non-mucinous cells. These histological findings help differentiate it from other vaginal cysts.

Müllerian cysts are another embryological remnant and typically found on the anterolateral vaginal wall. They are lined by secretory epithelium resembling a fallopian tube. They can occur anywhere in the vagina and usually contain mucus. They can only be differentiated from Gartner's duct cyst on histology.

Treatment: Complete surgical excision is the treatment of choice as marsupialisation has a higher rate of recurrence. Other treatments include surgical aspiration and injection of tetracycline solution, but are typically reserved for only small cysts.

Skene's Duct Cyst

Skene's glands are bilateral paraurethral glands derived from the urogenital sinus. They open into the external urethral meatus. Obstruction of a Skene's duct secondary to infection leads to cyst or abscess formation. This is often due to infection by *Neisseria gonorrhoeae* or *Chlamydia*.

These cysts can often be asymptomatic. Cysts larger than 2 cm can present with dysuria, recurrent urinary infection or voiding dysfunction. Abscesses are usually swollen and tender. Due to its location, it is essential to distinguish a Skene's duct cyst from a urethral diverticulum. Compression of a Skene's duct cyst won't lead to fluid extravasation, unlike a urethral diverticulum. MRI or translabial ultrasound and urethroscopy can be used to distinguish the two.

Women with small cysts can be offered conservative management with observation. Symptomatic larger cysts warrant complete surgical excision or marsupialisation, under antibiotic cover if infected.

Other Vaginal and Periurethral Lesions

Epithelial Inclusion Cysts

Epithelial inclusion cysts result from the mucosa becoming trapped in the submucosal area secondary to procedures such as episiotomy, vaginal wall repairs, and trauma including childbirth. These cysts are lined with squamous epithelium and contain keratin and sebaceous fluid. Large cysts can cause pain, and treatment is excision of the cyst.

Leiomyomas

Although rare, leiomyomas can present as an anterior vaginal wall mass. They originate from the smooth muscle of the urethra or the smooth muscle of the vaginal wall. Most are asymptomatic unless large, in which case symptoms are usually urinary. Surgical excision is the treatment of choice, and urethral reconstruction is likely to be needed with urethral leiomyomas. Malignant transformation is rare.

Urothelial Cyst

Urothelial cysts are uncommon and present as small cysts around the distal urethra. Lined by urothelium, the cause is thought to be surgical trauma. They are often asymptomatic. If symptomatic, surgical excision is indicated.

Conclusion

Vaginal, urethral and paraurethral benign cysts commonly present as swelling and the clinician should be able to ascertain the origin and nature of the cystic swelling. Imaging may be needed in some cases to establish the true nature of the lesion. Most of these cystic swellings can be managed in the ambulatory setting, even if they require catheterisation for short- term. Referral to a specialist should be considered in complex cases and if the diagnosis is in doubt.

Further Reading

Archer, R., Blackman, J., Stott, M., and Barrington, J. (2015). Urethral diverticulum. *Obstet. Gynaecol.* 17: 125–129.

Dolan, M.S., Hill, C., and Valea, F.A. (2017). Benign gynecologic lesions. In: *Comprehensive Gynecology* (eds. R.A.,.G. Lobo, G.M. Lentz and F.A. Valea), 371. Philadelphia: Elsevier.

Goh, J.T. (2004). A new classification for female genital tract fistula. *Aust. N. Z. J. Obstet. Gynaecol.* 44 (6): 502–504.

Stav K, Dwyer PL, Rosamilia A, Chao F, Urinary symptoms before and after female urethral diverticulectomy: Can we predict De Novo stress urinary incontinence? *J Urol* Sep 2008,17; PMD: 18804229.

Tsivian, M., Tsivian, A., Shreiber, L. et al. (2009). Female urethral diverticulum: a pathological insight. *Int. Urogynecol. J. Pelvic Floor Dysfunct.* 20 (8): 957–960.

10

Ambulatory Management of Childbirth Pelvic Floor Trauma

Khaled M.K. Ismail, Rasha Kamel, and Vladimir Kalis

Introduction

Annually, millions of women worldwide sustain trauma to the pelvic floor at the time of childbirth. A significant number of these women suffer short-term and sometimes long-term consequences, which can have a negative impact on both physical and emotional health, and also affect their quality of life. The burden of these complications is even greater when the age of the woman and the effect on her family is taken into account. In recent years, there has been a lot of focus on the prevention, assessment, and repair of childbirth-related pelvic floor trauma. There has been a plethora of evidence-based guidelines, quality improvement initiatives, and innovations and multidisciplinary training programmes devised to address these issues. Nevertheless, the focus has mainly been on intrapartum care with relatively less attention to the antenatal and postnatal periods.

There is wide global variation in maternity service provision and funding. Moreover, there are cultural differences that have an impact on several aspects of maternity care including shared norms, beliefs, and expectations. These factors will undoubtedly affect what services are being offered, how they are utilised, and what is being prioritised. Irrespective of the type or location of healthcare, postnatal services do not receive the same level of attention or funding as antenatal and intrapartum services. Furthermore, childbirth-related pelvic-floor trauma and its consequences do not receive the required level of attention because of the tendency to focus on pregnancy progress and foetal development. This, at least sometimes, translates to a significant number of women missing out on crucial information relating to current or previous childbirth pelvic floor trauma and how to mitigate the risk of complications in the short and long term. Although intrapartum management of pelvic-floor trauma is considered a core skill of any birth attendant, the management of its consequences requires specialised training.

Ambulatory Urology and Urogynaecology, First Edition. Edited by Abhay Rane and Ajay Rane.
© 2021 John Wiley & Sons Ltd. Published 2021 by John Wiley & Sons Ltd.

Women's pelvic floor pathology encompasses a wide spectrum of functional, anatomical and neurological problems, which may be associated with symptoms of bowel, urinary, and/or sexual dysfunction. Care for women with pelvic-floor trauma is, therefore, best delivered via a multidisciplinary approach.

Childbirth pelvic trauma and its complications can be addressed in the ambulatory care setting. This can include consultation, investigations, treatment, interventions, and sometimes rehabilitation services. We believe that this model of care should be utilised in the context of specialised postnatal clinics because it will ensure that women receive fast, effective, consistent, and evidence-based management without added pressure on other maternity services. We see the ambulatory care setting as an interface between primary and secondary care, receiving referrals from family physicians, community midwives, as well as hospital referrals. If the healthcare system allows, we believe women should be able to self-refer when plagued by a particular query or concern. In this chapter, we will cover the services and procedures that can be undertaken within an ambulatory service in relation to childbirth pelvic-floor trauma.

Perineal Wound Complications

In women undergoing vaginal delivery about 85% are known to sustain some form of perineal injury. The short-term sequelae of perineal injury include bleeding and pain, but may include wound complications such as infection, dehiscence and granulation tissue. Persistent pain after eight weeks postpartum occurs in about 22% of women and with about 20% experiencing dyspareunia.

Anal dysfunction such as faecal or flatus incontinence can occur with obstetric anal sphincter injuries (OASIs). In the long term, perineal trauma such as levator muscle avulsion has been postulated as risk factors for pelvic floor disorders such as pelvic organ prolapse and urinary incontinence.

Perineal Wound Infection

A two-iteration Delphi study of women who had previously sustained perineal trauma was undertaken to determine patient-reported outcomes for perineal trauma. The quality-improvement study demonstrated that the highest ranked outcome was fear of perineal wound infection and delay in wound healing.

There is growing evidence that the number of women reporting perineal wound dehiscence and infection in the community is increasing. A significant number of these wound breakdowns occur within the first two weeks of delivery. However, there are several issues that should be taken into account when discussing childbirth-related perineal wound infections. These include:

- In many healthcare settings there are no systems to track wound infection and dehiscence in the community and this has led to the wide disparity of prevalence from 0.59 to 13.5%.
- There is lack of perineal-wound validated screening tools that can be used in the community or primary care for early identification of infection.
- Disparity exists between clinically suspected and microbiologically confirmed perineal wound infection.
- Wide variation in the management of wound infection and dehiscence.

Perineal wound infection and dehiscence can have serious consequences on a woman's general health and quality of life. These problems include persistent pain and discomfort at the perineal wound site, urinary and bowel problems, and dyspareunia, as well as psychological and psychosexual issues from perceived or altered body image. The most serious complication that can arise is systemic sepsis. It is imperative, therefore, that women with suspected perineal infection are reviewed urgently. Women who have problems with their wound in the form of increasing pain, excessive or offensive discharge, pyrexia, feeling generally unwell, swelling of the wound, or evidence of wound dehiscence should have an urgent assessment.

There is a paucity of validated tools for the objective assessment of perineal wounds for the early detection and follow-up of wound infection. Until a more specific tool is available, we recommend the use of the REEDA score (Table 10.1) for perineal wound assessment. The REEDA tool assesses Redness (R), Edema (E), Ecchymosis (bruising) (E), Discharge (D) and approximation of the perineal wound edges (A). Its scientific merit relies upon taking precise measurements and providing objective descriptive data to assess the condition of the wound over a period of time.

If a wound infection is suspected, microbiological swabs should be taken from the perineal wound area and the woman should be prescribed appropriate broad-spectrum antibiotics. We recommend that the antibiotic regimen discussed and agreed upon with the local microbiology team is in line with unit policy. The prescribed antibiotics should be reviewed once the swab results are available. Further follow-up appointments will depend on the severity of infection, presence of wound breakdown, and general maternal condition. In general, it will be appropriate for the woman to be seen in the clinic weekly for the first two to three weeks. With each visit, an objective assessment of the wound condition using REEDA score should be performed and documented. Once the infection is cleared and the wound has healed, it would be prudent to arrange a follow-up visit after 8–12 weeks or even later, to check for any long-term complications such as perineal pain or dyspareunia.

Table 10.1 The REEDA score.

Score	Redness	Edema	Ecchymosis	Discharge	Approximation
0	None	None	None	None	Closed
1	Mild Less than 0.5 cm from each side of the wound edges	Mild Less than 1 cm from each side of the wound edges	Mild Less than 1 cm from each side of the wound edges	Serum	Skin separation 3 mm or less
2	Moderate 0.5 cm to 1 cm from each side of the wound edges	Moderate 1 to 2 cm from each side of the wound edges	Moderate 1 to 2 cm from each side of the wound edges	Serosanguinous	Skin and subcutaneous fat separation
3	Severe More than 1 cm from each side of the wound edges	Severe More than 2 cm from each side of the wound edges	Severe More than 2 cm from each side of the wound edges	Purulent	Skin and subcutaneous fat and fascial layer separation
Total				Overall score = +	

Dehiscence

Wound dehiscence is frequently preceded by or occurs in association with wound infection. This breakdown can involve the whole wound or only part of it. There is a wide variation in how a wound dehiscence is managed. Some favour expectant management; however, it can take up to 12–16 weeks for the wound to heal by secondary intention. The evidence for the management of such a complication is currently weak; nevertheless, it favours wound re-suturing 24–48 hours after appropriate antibiotic cover. The latter policy seems to be associated with a reduction in the time required for wound healing and improved satisfaction with the outcome after the wound has healed. In view of the negative impact of expectant management, we strongly recommend that women are counselled and given a choice about both management options so that they can make an informed choice. Re-suturing a dehisced wound will require anaesthesia for wound debridement and can be done as a day-care procedure under antibiotic cover in the absence of sepsis. An ambulatory clinic can identify complications, initiate treatment, provide counselling about management options, and follow up women after re-suturing and those opting for expectant management.

Granulation Tissue

When a wound heals by secondary intention, granulation tissue may form to bridge the gap between the wound edges. Less commonly, it can also form after wound healing by primary intention. Women tend to be referred with what is thought to be a skin tag, an area that is friable or bleeds easily when touched, or a persistent and excessive discharge. In almost all cases, the excessive granulation tissue can be chemically cauterised in the outpatient setting using silver nitrate. Sometimes more than one treatment is required.

Superficial Dyspareunia Following Childbirth

It is reported that 17–23% of women continue to experience superficial dyspareunia at three months after delivery and 10–14% at 12 months. In some studies, rates of 62 and 31% were reported for three and six months postnatal respectively. In view of the risk of such a problem triggering more complex psychosexual disorders, it is important that they are dealt with promptly, sensitively, and efficiently. The ambulatory set-up provides a suitable environment for this because women would be seen away from both obstetrics and gynaecology outpatient environments where they can be given more time and also have their problem assessed by a specialist.

The cause of superficial dyspareunia following childbirth can be physical and/ or psychological. One of the physical causes of superficial dyspareunia following perineal trauma or episiotomy is scar tissue at the introitus, particularly over the area of the fourchette (posterior commissure). This can result from excessive scar tissue formation or poor anatomical repair of the perineal tear. Typically, a thin band of scar tissue or a web of skin at the introitus can be seen on examination by parting the labia and slightly stretching the area of the fourchette. This web of skin or scar tissue will be very tender to touch on digital examination and during intercourse. Some women complain that it splits and bleeds during penetration. It is not uncommon for this problem to be missed on general inspection of the labia.

Conservative approaches, including the use of vaginal dilators, vibrators, and perineal massage have been reported to provide relief of symptoms in a minority of patients. The majority of women, however, will require a procedure to release or remove this area of scarring. A modified Fenton's procedure can be performed as an outpatient procedure under local anaesthesia. One of the main benefits of undertaking the procedure under local anaesthesia is the conscious pain mapping prior to surgery. The procedure follows the same concept as Fenton's, which involves a vertical incision, dissection of underlying scar tissue, followed by closure of the incision horizontally (Table 10.2). It is important to avoid overzealous dissection and the recommendation is to use fine fast absorbing polyglactin suture and a continuous technique for closure in two layers, to reduce the tension on the skin stitches.

Obstetric Anal Sphincter Injuries

Third- and fourth-degree perineal tears are collectively known as OASIs. This section will not cover the prevention, identification, or primary repair of OASIs but rather the management of women who have had this type of injury, in an ambulatory centre.

OASI Primary Repair and Follow-Up

It is good clinical practice that women who sustain OASIs have a follow-up appointment in a dedicated clinic at 12 weeks postnatally. During that visit we recommend the following:

- Take a detailed bowel history exploring the timing of the symptoms in relation to the OASIs. Using a bowel control, symptom-specific questionnaire can be of value in assessing the degree of anal dysfunction.
- Use the faecal incontinence severity index (FISI) and Faecal Incontinence Quality of Life assessment tools to improve the objective assessment (see Table 10.3).

Table 10.2 Steps of a modified Fenton procedure.

Band of scar tissue at the introitus part on parting the labia and very tender to touch	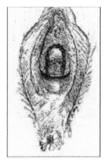
Vertical incision	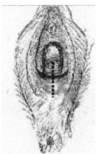
Dissection of underlying scar tissue	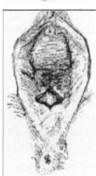
Repaired across in two layers using continuous 3/0 polyglactin suture	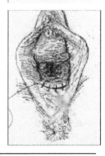

Source: Modified from Chandru et al. (2010).

Table 10.3   Faecal incontinence severity index.

	Never	Rarely	Sometimes	Usually	Always
a) Solid	0	1	2	3	4
b) Liquid	0	1	2	3	4
c) Gas	0	1	2	3	4
d) Wears pad	0	1	2	3	4
e) Lifestyle alteration	0	1	2	3	4

- Perform a clinical examination including checking the neurological function of sacral segments, such as the anal wink reflex.
- Assess the women's ability to perform correct and effective pelvic floor muscle training and discuss physiotherapy referral if required.
- Give the woman the opportunity to ask questions about her birth and trauma.
- Perform an endoanal ultrasound of the anal sphincter complex ± manometry.
- Discuss the short and long-term implications of the trauma and counsel her about mode of delivery for future births However, this will have to be reviewed with any future pregnancy if there is any change in her bowel symptoms.

Further investigations, follow-up, and multidisciplinary involvement will need to be tailored to the woman's needs.

Ultrasonography

Assessment of the internal and external anal sphincter by means of ultrasonography can be performed using an endoanal ultrasound (EAUS) or exo-anally using trans perineal ultrasound scanning (TPUS). Colorectal surgeons traditionally use endoanal ultrasonography, however, the availability of high-resolution volume sonography and tomographic ultrasound has made the diagnostic accuracy of trans perineal scanning in identifying anal sphincter pathology very comparable to that of endoanal ultrasound. TPUS also has the added advantages of cost saving, patient acceptability, and the avoidance of internal stretch of the anal canal and sphincters. With volume sonography, a volume is acquired with subsequent multiplanar and tomographic ultrasound imaging (TUI) sub-analysis. For TUI, an anal sphincter defect is defined as a defect of 30° or greater in the circumference of the external anal sphincter in at least two of three slices for EAUS or four of six slices for TPUS. Comparative studies of EAUS and 3D TPUS suggest good agreement. A step-by-step practical guide on how to perform and interpret a TPUS for the assessment of the anal sphincters is listed in Box 10.1.

Box 10.1 Technique of TPUS for the Assessment of the Anal Sphincters

1) Patient in lithotomy position.
2) Place vaginal probe vertically at the introitus on the posterior fourchette.
3) Start scanning in the sagittal plane till the anal canal is identified.
4) Without tilting, rotate by 90° to scan in the coronal plane. Alternatively, the probe is horizontally placed on the perineum and gradually inclined until the best view of the sphincters is achieved.
5) Care should be taken not to exert any pressure on the perineum, which may distort the anatomy.
6) The hypo-echogenic ring, representing the internal anal sphincter (IAS) encircling the echogenic irregularity of the anal mucosa and the completeness of the outer hyper-echogenic ring reflecting the external anal sphincter is obtained.
7) In 3D TPUS examinations, describe defects of the external anal sphincter by a clock-face notation or degrees as in measurements of angles in the coronal plane. On applying TUI volume sub analysis, an anal sphincter defect is defined as a defect of 30° or greater in the circumference of the external anal sphincter in at least four of six slices (two of three slices for EAUS) (Figure 10.5).
8) If IAS is torn, it retracts posteriorly creating the 'half-moon' sign.

Anorectal Manometry

Anorectal manometry is used for the functional assessment of the anal canal and rectum. The anal sphincter pressures, rectal sensation, and anorectal reflexes are measured using a number of pressure sensors mounted on a narrow balloon-tipped catheter inserted into the rectum. The parameters measured include:

- Anal canal resting pressure, which is generated by the resting tone of the IAS (normal range 61–163 cm H_2O).
- Voluntary anal squeeze pressure generated by the external anal sphincter contraction (normal range 50–181 cm H_2O).
- Involuntary anal squeeze pressure generated by asking the woman to cough to assess the external anal sphincter reflex (normal range 50–100 cm H_2O).

Mode of Birth in Pregnancies Subsequent to OASIs

Following OASIs, women should be counselled about the mode of birth in subsequent pregnancies. Current guidelines recommend that women who have neither bowel symptoms subsequent to their OASIs nor significant abnormality on ultrasonographic evaluation of the sphincters or anorectal manometry be offered a vaginal birth. There are fairly good levels of evidence to support this recommendation. In contrast, women who do not fulfil the aforementioned criteria should be offered an elective caesarean section in subsequent births, but the evidence in support of the latter recommendation is not robust.

In women who attend for follow up after OASIs and undergo anatomical and functional assessment of the anorectal complex, there is no reason that this discussion cannot be initiated at that time. This approach will give women the opportunity to plan future pregnancies based on clinical information specific to them. Although ultrasound findings should not change overtime, the woman's symptoms or anorectal manometry might. We, therefore, recommend that a detailed assessment of the woman's bowel function should be undertaken again during the antenatal period of any future pregnancy and the mode of birth re-discussed before a final recommendation is made. Women who did not have investigations performed during the follow-up of their OASIs will need to have these performed during the antenatal period of their subsequent pregnancy. An ambulatory set-up provides a one-stop setting where investigations, results, and counselling can take place with the aim to improve efficiency and reduce a woman's anxiety.

Levator Ani Muscle Avulsion

Pelvic floor disorders, urinary incontinence, and pelvic organ prolapse have been identified as important long-term complications of perineal trauma. Apart from the neurological damage and stretching of pelvic floor muscles in vaginal deliveries, the avulsion injury sustained to pelvic floor muscles is attributed as an important causative factor in pelvic floor disorders.

Levator avulsion (LA) is the detachment of the pubovisceral muscle (PVM) component of the levator ani muscle from its insertion into the pubic bone. There is wide variation in the reported incidence of avulsion injury, which ranges from 13 to 36% after the first birth. The risk is significantly higher following operative vaginal birth especially with forceps. The difference in incidence is also contributed to by the variation in the method and timing of diagnosis. LA can be complete or partial and either unilateral or bilateral. Although partial avulsions are more likely to improve over time, they are still associated with subjective and objective pelvic floor dysfunction. Palpation of the site of insertion of the PVM is sometimes recommended as a method of screening for LA, however, the diagnostic accuracy of this method relies on the skill of the examiner and the presence of an intact side to act as a reference. Nonetheless, natural variation in PVM insertions is a real limitation to this technique. Therefore, accurate diagnosis relies on imaging techniques, mainly in the form of 3D ultrasonography or magnetic-resonance imaging (MRI). For this reason, the diagnosis tends to be made a long time after birth. Good agreement between MRI and 3D TPUS has been reported with the ultrasound assessment being more reproducible, more convenient and more cost-effective. The TPUS assessment for LA should be undertaken upon pelvic muscle contraction for better tissue enhancement and with a volume acquisition angle of at least 70°. On TUI sub-analysis, LA is diagnosed when abnormal insertion is detected in three central slices or with a levatorurethral-gap (LUG) of >2.5 cm (Figures 10.1–10.4).

Although LA is known to increase a woman's long-term risk of prolapse, there is currently no policy or recommendation for routine screening even in high-risk women (e.g., after forceps deliveries or births complicated by OASIs). If there is a clinical need to confirm or refute the possibility of an LA, the presence of clinical expertise and an imaging facility within the ambulatory clinic is beneficial. At present, there are no effective surgical interventions for the repair of LA. There does, however, seem to be potential benefits in structured antenatal pelvic floor muscle exercises and alteration of avoidable risk factors such as obesity and constipation to reduce the individual woman's likelihood of developing significant pelvic floor disorders in the future.

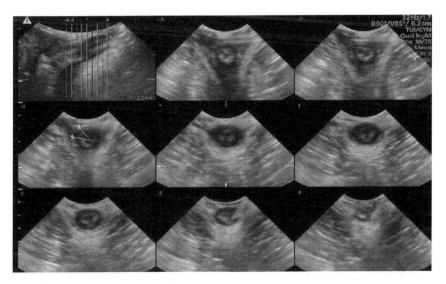

Figure 10.1 TUI sub-analysis of a 3D volume TPUS of a normally attached levator ani upon muscle contraction.

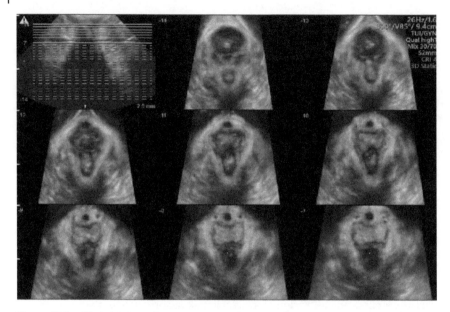

Figure 10.2 3D Axial view of a unilateral right sided levator avulsion.

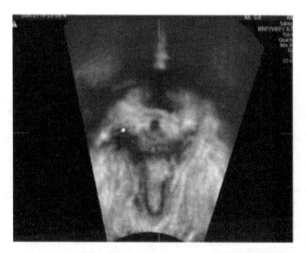

Figure 10.3 TUI sub-analysis of a 3D volume TPUS of a unilateral right sided levator avulsion with a LUG of 27.9 mm.

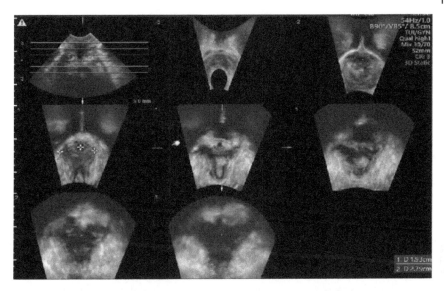

Figure 10.4   TUI sub-analysis of a 3D volume TPUS showing bilateral Levator avulsion.

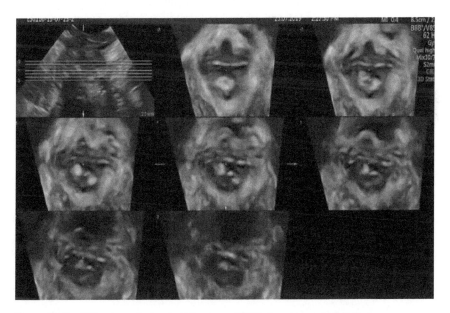

Figure 10.5   TUI sub-analysis of a 3D volume TPUS showing an EAS defect.

Conclusion

Perineal trauma after childbirth can pose significant physical and psychological morbidity. A dedicated centre in the ambulatory set-up, which provides consultation alongside imaging modalities and the ability to perform day-care surgical procedures, will be the way forward in caring for these women.

Further Reading

Chandru, S., Nafee, T., Ismail, K. et al. (2010). Evaluation of Modified Fenton procedure for persistent superficial dyspareunia following childbirth. *Gynecol Surg* 7: 245–248. https://doi.org/10.1007/s10397-009-0501-7.

Dietz, H.P. (2018). Exoanal imaging of the anal sphincters. *J. Ultrasound Med.* 37: 263–280. https://doi.org/10.1002/jum.14246.

Dudley, L.M., Kettle, C., and Ismail, K.M. (2013). Secondary suturing compared to non-suturing for broken down perineal wounds following childbirth. *Cochrane Database Syst. Rev.*: 9. https://doi.org/10.1002/14651858.CD008977.pub2.

Hiller, L., Radley, S., Mann, C.H. et al. (2002). Development and validation of a questionnaire for the assessment of bowel and lower urinary tract symptoms in women. *BJOG An Int. J. Obstet. Gynaecol.* 109: 413–423. https://doi.org/10.1111/j.1471-0528.2002.01147.x.

Ismail, K.M.K., Kettle, C., Macdonald, S.E. et al. (2013). Perineal assessment and repair longitudinal study (PEARLS): a matched-pair cluster randomized trial. *BMC Med* 11 https://doi.org/10.1186/1741-7015-11-209.

Laine, K., Rotvold, W., and Staff AC (2013). Are obstetric anal sphincter ruptures preventable?- large and consistent rupture rate variations between the Nordic countries and between delivery units in Norway. *Acta Obstet. Gynecol. Scand.* 92: 94–100. https://doi.org/10.1111/aogs.12024.

Royal College of Obstetricians & Gynaecologists (2015). The Management of Third- and Fouth-Degree Perineal Tears: green-top Guideline No. 29. *R. Coll. Obstet. Gynaecol.* 29: 1–11.

11

Teaching and Training in Urogynaecology

Ajay Rane

Urogynaecologists specialise in the female pelvic organs and their supporting structures. This involves treating pelvic floor disorders including pelvic organ prolapse, bladder and bowel dysfunction, incontinence, pelvic or bladder pain, and fistulas. These specialists are surgically trained and many will also be skilled in performing ultrasound. Urogynaecologists divide their time across outpatient clinics, the operating theatre, outpatient procedures such as cystoscopy or urodynamics, and ultrasound scanning. This work can be performed in the public or private sector.

The practice of urogynaecology allows for a mix of clinical medicine, imaging, and surgery. Many women are either too embarrassed to address their issues or see them as a normal function of childbirth and ageing. The practice of urogynaecology allows women to successfully manage what are often chronic issues and regain their quality of life. By focusing on a particular area of gynaecology, subspecialists are able to offer patients a higher level of expertise and training in the management of pelvic floor dysfunction.

Role of the Generalist Gynaecologist in Urogynaecology

The general gynaecologist is trained in the management of pelvic floor dysfunction and can manage many of the common urogynaecological presentations. The general gynaecologist is often the first point of contact after the general practitioner. When management has failed or is beyond the expertise of the generalist, referral to a subspecialist is recommended. Complex cases, such as women who have had previous surgeries or mesh complications, are best managed by a subspecialist whose training and experience in the area may translate to better patient

Ambulatory Urology and Urogynaecology, First Edition. Edited by Abhay Rane and Ajay Rane.
© 2021 John Wiley & Sons Ltd. Published 2021 by John Wiley & Sons Ltd.

outcomes. The following is a summary of the role and qualifications of a generalist gynaecologist in various countries:

Australia

The general gynaecologist in Australia will have been signed off for basic vaginal surgery (anterior and posterior repair), intermediate vaginal surgery (vaginal hysterectomy), and minor perineal surgery. The expectation prior to sign-off is that the candidate will have completed 20 basic surgeries and 20 intermediate surgeries, which are guides and not mandatory numbers. While there is no sign-off assessment for continence procedures, the logbook recommendation is the performance of five continence surgeries during training. It is also expected that trainees will have spent at least 100 hours in gynaecology outpatient clinics.

The Royal Australian and New Zealand College of Obstetrics and Gynaecology (RANZCOG) introduced Advanced Training Modules in 2019. There are two compulsory and four optional modules. One of the optional modules pertains to urogynaecology – the pelvic floor disorders module. This can be undertaken over a 12–24 month period during advanced training and should include a minimum of 45 urogynaecology theatre sessions and 45 urogynaecology outpatient clinic sessions per 12 months. Requirements for this module include a logbook, presentation at morbidity and mortality meetings, and presentation of an audit of pelvic floor treatment outcomes. The suggested numbers for logbook procedures include: urinary stress incontinence procedures (10), vaginal hysterectomy (10), anterior and/or posterior vaginal repair (20), post-hysterectomy vaginal vault suspension procedures (5), urodynamic studies (10) and cystoscopy (20).

United Kingdom (UK)

The Royal College of Obstetricians and Gynaecologists (RCOG) offer advanced training skills modules (ATSM) in the final two years of obstetrics and gynaecology. This training allows trainees to develop the skills required to practice in various subspecialty areas as part of a generalist job with a particular focus or interest. The relevant module is Urogynaecology and Vaginal Surgery (UGVS). An optional laparoscopic urogynaecology module is also available, but can only be undertaken after completion of the UGVS ATSM or concurrently with it (i.e., it cannot be undertaken as a stand-alone module). On completion of the ATSM, it would be expected that a trainee would be competent in: anterior repair, diagnostic cystourethroscopy ± biopsy, mid-urethral tape (retropubic or trans-obturator approach), posterior repair ± perineorrhaphy and vaginal hysterectomy.

United States of America (USA)

In the USA, there are 241 obstetrics and gynaecology residency programmes (1288 spots available). These programmes are all individualised and some have more exposure to urogynaecology than others. On completion of residency, a generalist obstetrician and gynaecologist (OBGYN) would be able to perform a vaginal hysterectomy, uterine and vaginal vault suspension procedures, and prolapse repairs.

Formal Urogynaecological Training by Country

Australia

Training in Australia is managed by RANZCOG. The training is three years in duration at a minimum of two prospectively approved training sites. RANZCOG trainees can undertake up to one year of subspecialty training as part of their advanced training for their fellowship of the College. The first year of training must be undertaken on a full-time basis. Selection is via a process of online application including covering letter, personal statement, curriculum vitae, and three references. Suitable applicants will then be invited to attend a panel interview.

Requirements for training include maintenance of a logbook, written examination, research project, formative review (at 3 and 9 months each year) and summative appraisals (at 6 and 12 months each year). Multisource feedback is also sought in the first year of training.

Minimum numbers are set for anti-incontinence procedures and reconstructive procedures (100 of each). Attendance at urogynaecology lectures, tutorials, demonstrations, and conferences is also expected.

The examination is of 3.25 hours duration and consists of 10 short answer questions.

Some procedures are considered compulsory and need to be formally assessed and signed off by a supervisor. There are two categories – generic procedural, of which there are 8, and surgical procedural, of which there are 11.

Some time spent during training in an overseas unit is considered desirable.

The following objectives are from the handbook for the certification in urogynaecology:

It is expected that the subspecialist in urogynaecology will:

- Demonstrate a detailed knowledge of:
  - The embryology and anatomy of the pelvis, the pelvic musculature, and the pelvic viscera

- The physiology of urinary and faecal control
- The pathology of abnormal urinary and faecal control
- Neurotransmission and the pharmacology of drugs acting directly and indirectly on the lower urinary tract
- Have a basic knowledge of:
  - Imaging of upper and lower urinary tracts
  - The design and statistical analysis of clinical trials
  - The function of urodynamic equipment
- Have an extensive personal experience in the assessment of patients with lower urinary tract disorders by:
  - Clinical assessment
  - Urodynamic assessment
  - Cystourethroscopy
  - Organ imaging
- Have a clinical competence in the following:
  - The medical and surgical management of pelvic floor dysfunction including genital tract prolapse
  - The surgical and medical management of lower urinary tract dysfunction
  - The long-term care of patients with intractable incontinence
  - Organisation of community care of the incontinent community assessment procedures liaison with nursing and general practitioner services

United Kingdom

In Britain, candidates for urogynaecology training complete subspecialty training as the final two years of a seven-year general obstetrics and gynaecology (O&G) training programme.

Eligibility

To enter subspecialty training, there is a need to fulfil one of the following criteria:

1) Hold a UK national training number or equivalent, including successful completion of clinical training to ST5 or ST6 level, confirmed by outcome 1 in most recent Annual Review of Competency Progression (ARCP) or equivalent, and have passed the Part 3 MRCOG.
2) Or hold a UK Certificate of Completion of Training (CCT) or Certificate of Eligibility for Specialist Registration (CESR) and be on the UK specialist register in obstetrics and gynaecology (O&G).
3) Be a European Economic Area or non-UK applicant who is listed on the UK specialist register in O&G.

Training Requirements

The programme consisting of eight modules and two courses: the ATSM course (same as for general urogynaecology) and a leadership and management course. Competency is required in the following objective structured assessment of technical skills (OSATs) for subspecialty trainees: colposuspension, cystoscopy, midurethral sling, posterior repair, sacro-colpopexy, sacrospinous fixation, urodynamics, vaginal hysterectomy, anterior repair, laparoscopic sacro-colpopexy (optional module only), and laparoscopic sacro-hysteropexy (optional module only).

There are also eight mini clinical evaluation exercises (Mini-CEXs), eight case-based discussions (CbDs), and team observation forms at least twice a year. Competency in clinical governance include patient safety, audit, risk management, and quality improvement. Trainees must maintain a logbook.

United States of America

In the United States, training in urogynaecology is called the Female Pelvic Medicine and Reconstructive Surgery (FPMRS) Fellowship. The subspecialty certification has been available since 2011.

Eligibility

The fellowship involves a three-year commitment after completion of Obstetrics and Gynaecology residency or a two-year commitment after completing a urology residency. Some residency programmes provide more FPMRS exposure and training than others. The fellowship application process occurs during the third year of residency and hence it can be difficult for some residents to have the requisite exposure to this field prior to the application deadlines. All accredited FPMRS fellowship programmes require candidates to undertake research to develop and defend a thesis.

Application is through a standardised process via the Electronic Residency Application Service (ERAS). Applicants must ensure they meet all programme prerequisites and institutional policies regarding eligibility for appointment prior to ranking a programme through the National Resident Matching Program. Candidates are then selected for interview. Candidates who have done research and attended the American Urogynaecologic Society (AUGS) annual meetings will be considered highly. It is also recommended to seek mentorship and a letter of recommendation from a well-connected faculty member. Candidates also need to apply to participating programmes and apply to the institutions they are interested in. The interview process is expensive and it is typically recommended that candidates interview at approximately 10 programmes. Although the cost is variable, candidates should roughly budget US$4500 to US$9500. The vast majority of this money is spent on travel because most applicants will travel to 10 or more interviews.

Training Requirements

The curriculum varies from hospital to hospital and needs to be approved by the Accreditation Council for Graduate Medical Education (ACGME). The ACGME reviews each programme and accredit each if they can demonstrate that trainees have adequate training time to develop the following skills: (i) demonstration of competence in patient care, medical knowledge, practice-based learning and improvement, interpersonal and communication skills, professionalism, and systems-based practice competency requirements; and, (ii) completion of a scholarly paper or quality improvement project. The Review Committee will annually review major components of the programme curriculum to monitor compliance with these requirements. Further information on the milestones required during training can be found at: www.acgme.org/Portals/0/PDFs/Milestones/FemalePelvicMedicinean dReconstructiveSurgeryMilestones.pdf?ver=2016-04-04-143644-683.

An example of a possible curriculum follows:

Fellows will learn how to evaluate, manage, and treat patients with primary pelvic organ prolapse and bladder control problems, as well as complex pelvic floor disorders, including urethral diverticulum, vesicovaginal or rectovaginal fistula, and pelvic floor myofascial pain.

Fellows will be trained to perform the full scope of surgical procedures, including:

- Laparoscopic Sacro colpopexy
- Robotic Sacro colpopexy
- Vaginal hysterectomy
- Vaginal apical suspension procedures
- Slings
- Bulking injection procedures
- Sacral neuromodulation
- Peripheral nerve stimulation
- Vaginal electrical stimulation

Low-Resource Countries – FIGO Recommendations

The International Federation of Gynaecology and Obstetrics (FIGO) recognises that not every country will be able to provide trainees with the resources or facilities in which to achieve all of the goals of training that are set out for achievement in highly resourced countries. The FIGO Task Force has therefore created guidelines for resident/general physician training to suggest minimum standards for urogynaecology services for women in low–moderate resource countries. The requirements follow:

Knowledge (both specifically and broadly) should include *at least* the following topics by the end of training:

- Trauma and congenital anomalies that result in incontinence
- Voiding dysfunction and urinary retention
- Urinary incontinence types and assessment
- Overactive bladder
- Painful bladder syndrome/interstitial cystitis
- Urinary tract infection
- Lower urinary and intestinal tract fistulae
- Pelvic pain syndrome
- Pelvic organ prolapse
- Childbirth – related pelvic floor trauma
- Urethral lesions, i.e. diverticula
- Effects of surgery and irradiation on the lower urinary and intestinal tracts and pelvic floor function
- Urinary disorders in pregnancy (including infections and incontinence)
- Evaluation and care of the elderly with pelvic floor disorders
- Lesions of the central nervous system affecting urinary and faecal control and pelvic floor function
- Disorders of the lower intestinal tract including difficult defecation, faecal incontinence, and rectal prolapse
- Obstetric anal sphincter injury
- Emotional and behavioural disorders affecting the pelvic floor and lower urinary and intestinal tract function
- Urinary disorders of childhood
- Pelvic floor disorders in the physically and mentally challenged individual
- Sexually transmitted diseases
- Effect of hormone deficiency states on the pelvic floor
- Urinary problems secondary to medical conditions and drugs
- Sexual dysfunction and coital incontinence
- Vulvar disorders
- Principles of evidence-based medicine, epidemiology, and critical appraisal of urogynaecologic research
- Electronic and non-electronic urodynamics studies.

Emerging Nations/Low-Resource Settings

Many low-resource settings are unable to provide training that meets the FIGO requirements. It can be quite difficult for doctors in low-income countries to not only access appropriate training in their own countries but also abroad. It can actually be quite difficult for residents in first-world countries to get into subspecialty training in their own countries. The obstacles for foreigners are often substantially higher. An example of a surgeon who is actively working to train surgeons in low-resource settings is Dr Stephen Jeffrey.

Dr Stephen Jeffrey – South Africa

Dr Stephen Jeffery is a urogynaecologist in South Africa. He received his accreditation at the Royal College in London. He was the first gynaecologist in South Africa to have received specialised training and accreditation in pelvic surgery and reconstruction. He was awarded his subspecialty degree with distinction. He is also president of the South African Urogynaecology Association. In this role, Dr Jeffery has been instrumental in formalising the accreditation of urogynaecology as a subspecialty in South Africa. He has trained surgeons from the USA, UK, Ghana, Pakistan, India, United Arab Emirates, Kenya, Philippines, Germany, Nepal, Mozambique, and Mauritius both in Cape Town and in their own countries.

Use of Technology and Simulation in Training

Laparoscopic surgery lends itself to simulation. From the basic box trainer to multi-million-dollar computer simulation software, similar to flight simulators, trainees can practice their laparoscopic surgical skills. Some of the more advanced simulators also have haptics, which give feedback to the hands when an object is 'touched' on the screen.

Vaginal surgeries can be difficult for the trainee to grasp due to the confined operating space and sometimes 'blind' operation (e.g., sacrospinous fixation). The operating surgeon has command of the operation while the trainee initially holds retractors. It can be difficult to transition from the assistant to the primary operator. Technology has not left vaginal surgeons behind however. The VITOM® – Video Telescopic Operating Telescope developed by Karl Storz, allows for video recording of operations for teaching purposes. The trainee can follow on a screen what the operator is doing. This technology can also be used to 'live-stream' operations to another room in the hospital (with patient consent) so that multiple doctors can observe without compromising sterility. With the addition of video recording technology in the theatre, the operating surgeon can also speak to the observing team.

There are also multiple resources available on the Internet with surgical videos and training modules. Often fee-based membership of these sites is required. Some of these websites have a particular gynaecology or urogynaecological focus. For example, the International Academy of Pelvic Surgery has modules on sling procedures, reconstructive procedures of the lower urinary tract, ureteral surgery, surgical correction of pelvic organ prolapse, surgery for posterior pelvic floor abnormalities, surgical management of mesh complications after sling procedures, and mesh prolapse repairs, challenging cases in urogynaecology. Their website is https://academyofpelvicsurgery.com/video-library.

Research

The highest goal of medicine is to practice an evidenced-based model of care. Urogynaecology, being a relatively new field, data is often lacking but research opportunities are many in this area. The gold standard for treatment for many common conditions, such as interstitial cystitis, are still being investigated and developed. Many training programmes have a research component and there is scope for more research. Fellows should be encouraged to perform research in areas of particular interests to them, and doctors with an interest in research would be welcomed into the speciality.

The Mesh Saga

Currently, all vaginal mesh products have been removed from the market – as of May 2019. Vaginal mesh for urogynaecological procedures was first approved in the United States in 1996. Twelve years later (2008), the Therapeutic Goods Administration (TGA) in Australia received the first adverse-events reports.Two years later (2010), the US Food and Drug Administration (FDA) issued a safety communication, recommending that surgeons consider further specialised training before inserting mesh while the TGA was investigating the reported adverse events and consulting with an expert panel. The United States, Australia, and New Zealand committees were all emphasising the need for informed consent prior to insertion of mesh, so that patients understood that mesh was permanent, not without complications, and that these complications could not always be resolved with or without further surgery.

Over the following few years, further reports emerged on the complications associated with vaginal mesh and more investigations began. The literature reported conflicting information on success rates of mesh. By 2011, the FDA had updated their communication to advise that the evidence did not support the use of posterior compartment mesh. The communication also advised that, although anterior compartment mesh efficacy had some weight of evidence to support it, adverse events were not rare and, therefore, patients should be counselled appropriately prior to mesh insertion in addition to being advised that long-term data to support mesh was limited. Post-market surveillance was stepped up. In 2014, urogynaecological meshes were being withdrawn from the market amid increasing concerns about the potential for serious and life-altering complications. In 2015, reviews from multiple countries including Scotland, UK, the European Commission, Australia, and New Zealand were published. These resulted in the reclassification of vaginal mesh by the FDA in 2016 to Class III – a high risk device. Other countries followed suit in 2017. In the meantime, the PROSPECT study, a Scottish multi-centre trial showed no benefit of vaginal mesh over native tissue repair. This ultimately led to the withdrawal of all mesh by mid-2019. Class actions have been undertaken against manufacturer's and the outcome of these is awaited.

Initial success with the adoption of transvaginal insertion of slings for urinary stress incontinence soon led to their widespread acceptance as the gold standard treatment. There were also initial reports that mesh showed promise for the repair of pelvic organ prolapse. Many soon adopted it as the primary treatment for pelvic organ prolapse. Could the complications have been predicted? Manufacturers have been blamed for promoting the technology before results were available from randomised controlled trials. Was it the case that surgeons without appropriate training were adopting an industry-driven new technology as a primary prolapse surgery with the promise of a 'permanent solution' to prolapse? Should the procedure have been left to pelvic floor specialists, such as urogynaecologists? From current data, it is hard to know whether there is a subset of patients that would benefit from mesh – for example, recurrent anterior compartment prolapse in a non-smoker with a normal BMI. Could better case selection have prevented the current situation? Again, from current data, it is difficult to know. The fallout will continue and the answers to these questions may become evident with hindsight.

Training Status

The UK (RCOG) removed mesh procedures from their advanced training modules and subspecialty training modules in October 2018. Urethrotomy and 'stapled trans-anal resection procedure' were also removed. Sacrospinous fixation was added to the module at the same time.

When the Australian advanced training module was introduced in 2019, no vaginal mesh procedures were expected. The vaginal mesh saga has also led to investigation into mesh for sub-urethral slings. As of December 2017, RANZCOG have removed sub-urethral slings from the general training requirements for general obstetrics and gynaecology trainees in light of the difficulties in obtaining exposure and training for these procedures. Prior to this time, surgical competency in transvaginal tape was required. This followed a decision in December 2016 to reduce the requirement from 20 continence procedures to 5 and a change to the assessment of the procedure. The procedure could be signed off with some input or 'minimal input' from the assessor (i.e., the trainee no longer had to be competent to perform the procedure independently). The Australian advanced training module specifies that 10 surgical procedures for urinary stress incontinence are expected, but does not specify the mode of operation. A trainee completing the pelvic floor disorders advanced training module could continue to perform incontinence surgery after graduating provided they perform more than 20 such procedures each year to maintain competency. It is expected that auditing of this will follow. Mesh removal has become the province of the urogynaecologist and training courses now include procedures for mesh removal.

What can be learned from this?

Early adoption of technology without appropriate trials of efficacy can lead to long-term debilitating consequences for patients that may lead to poor quality of life. It behoves us all to question the rigour of research and trials before adopting new techniques and technologies.

Appropriate training is also important and those learning, should be taught by experienced operators.

In summary, urogynaecology is an expanding specialty that is progressing our knowledge of the female pelvic floor and exploring ways to face its challenges and conundrums.

Further Reading

Accreditation Council for Graduate Medical Education website (n.d.). www.acgme.org

Drutz, H.P. (2010). IUGA guidelines for training in female pelvic medicine and reconstructive pelvic surgery – updated guidelines 2010. *Int. Urogynecol. J.* 21: 1445–1453.

RANZCOG (2019). Certification in Urogynaecology. RANZCOG Training Program Handbook. Melbourne Australia. https://ranzcog.edu.au/Training/Subspecialist-Training/Current-Trainees-(4)/Training-Program-Handbooks.

RCOG (n.d.). ATSM urogynaecology and vaginal surgery. www.rcog.org.uk/en/careers-training/specialty-training-curriculum/atsms/atsms-pre-august-2019/atsm-urogynaecology-and-vaginal-surgery.

RCOG Urogynaecology Curriculum (2018). October. www.rcog.org.uk/en/careers-training/specialty-training-curriculum/subspecialty-training/urogynaecology-subspecialty-training.

Senate Community Affairs Committee Secretariat (2018). Number of women in Australia who have had transvaginal mesh implants and related matters. Parliamentary Report (28 March 2018). Senate Printing Unit, Parliament House, Canberra.

Stenchever, M.A., Rizk, D.E., Falconi, G., and Ortiz, O.C. (2009). FIGO guidelines for training residents and fellow in Urogynaecology female urology and female pelvic medicine and reconstructive surgery. *Int. J. Gyne. Obs.* 107 (3): 187–190.

Section III

Ambulatory Urology

Foreword

The concept of 'ambulatory care' is an evolving one, but as new systems and techniques are developed, urology is one of the surgical specialties that remains poised to best take advantage of these. Ambulatory urology encompasses not only surgical procedures with same-day discharge, but also outpatient attendances encompassing multiple tests and investigations in one visit.

In the drive for healthcare to be efficient, cost-effective, and timely for patients, urology units are now increasingly looking for new ways to deliver an 'ambulatory service.' So-called 'one-stop' clinics for the investigation of haematuria are now commonplace and increasingly similar models are being employed for assessment of possible prostate cancer and benign conditions such as lower urinary tract symptoms.

With advances in surgical technology, a very high proportion of urological operations are now completed as 'day-cases.' Just a few decades ago, ureteric stones were managed with open ureter lithotomy and an inpatient stay of several nights, today ureteric stones are treated with ureteroscopy and laser stone fragmentation and patients are normally discharged home within a few hours of leaving the operating theatre. The vast majority of penile and scrotal surgery is now considered ambulatory and new techniques such as Rezūm prostate surgery mean that a high proportion of urological pathologies have an ambulatory option for management. In the coming years we are likely to see increased usage of robot assisted laparoscopy as more surgeons are exposed to it during their training and more manufacturers enter the marketplace. Day-surgery robot-assisted prostatectomy is already a reality in some units, and this opens the door to ambulatory robot-assisted surgery one day becoming the rule, rather than the exception.

Jordan Durrant

12

Ambulatory Penile and Inguino-Scrotal Surgery

Ben Pullar

Background

Day-case or ambulatory surgery is now the standard-of-care for the majority of penile and inguino-scrotal procedures in modern urology. However, same-day discharge cannot be reliably achieved unless consideration is given to achieving this from the outset. In general, the patient should be aware of the nature of the procedure and the intention that they will be discharged home the same day. This starts at the initial clinic consultation and will continue through effective pre-assessment to the day of the procedure itself. Recovery and ward nursing staff are essential in delivering effective day case surgery with nurse-led discharge now becoming routine, following a clear post-operative plan from the operating surgeon.

Specific to surgical procedures, particular attention should be made to adequate post-operative analgesia, catheter management (if applicable), and meticulous haemostasis to avoid unnecessary re-admissions due to these preventable issues.

Individual Conditions and Procedures

Hydrocele

A hydrocele is an accumulation of fluid between the two layers (parietal and visceral) of the tunica vaginalis surrounding the testes. The diagnosis is made on clinical examination and it is important to differentiate a hydrocele from other causes of scrotal swelling. Examination will reveal a smooth, unilateral scrotal swelling with a palpable superior margin which trans illuminates. It is often difficult to palpate the underlying testes.

Ambulatory Urology and Urogynaecology, First Edition. Edited by Abhay Rane and Ajay Rane.
© 2021 John Wiley & Sons Ltd. Published 2021 by John Wiley & Sons Ltd.

The differential diagnosis of a unilateral scrotal swelling includes varicocele, hernia, epididymal cyst, infection (orchiditis), or tumour.

Diagnosis is supported by ultrasound, which will both confirm the diagnosis and confirm that the underlying testes are normal.

Surgical management of a hydrocele is indicated if symptomatic. Small hydrocoeles or larger, asymptomatic hydroceles can be safely managed conservatively.

Hydrocele repair performed as a day case is well established. However, in older patients or men with a large hydrocele in which a drain is placed post operatively, an overnight admission may be warranted. Paediatric hydroceles are managed differently with a groin incision and ligation of a patent processes vaginalis. They are almost always performed as a day-case procedure. There are three options for surgical management of an adult hydrocele. Definitive surgical repair is with either a Jaboulay or Lord's technique. The Lord's procedure is suitable for small and medium sized hydroceles. It involves plication of the hydrocele sac. Larger hydrocoeles may be managed with the Jaboulay procedure in which the hydrocele sac is excised. Both procedures can be complicated by recurrence or haematoma formation. A drain insertion may be used for larger hydroceles to prevent haematoma accumulation.

Hydrocele aspiration (with or without sclerotherapy) may be reserved for a patient deemed unfit to undergo any general anaesthesia (GA) procedure, but accepting the high recurrence rates associated with it and the risk of haematoma.

Varicocele

Varicocele is defined as a dilatation of the pampiniform plexus of veins in the spermatic cord. It is common and estimated to affect 15% of the general male population. It is seen much more commonly in men being investigated for both primary and secondary infertility.

Varicoceles develop from incompetent valves in the spermatic veins resulting in retrograde blood flow and engorgement of and subsequent dilatation of the veins in the pampiniform plexus. It is more common on the left side due the higher pressures within the left testicular vein owing to the acute angle at which it enters the left renal vein. (This is in contrast to the oblique angle at which the right-side testicular vein enters the inferior vena cava (IVC), resulting in lower pressure on the right side).Most varicoceles are asymptomatic but if large may cause scrotal discomfort. They are commonly identified as part of the investigation of male subfertility. The link between varicoceles and infertility is thought to result from a loss of the countercurrent heat exchange mechanism that exists such that scrotal temperatures are lower than the rest of the body. The resulting rise in scrotal temperatures results in impaired spermatogenesis.

Diagnosis is on clinical examination and graded according to size. It is classically described as 'a bag of worms'. Diagnosis is confirmed with scrotal ultrasound.

Treatment of a varicocele should be considered in sympomatic cases. The treatment of varicocele for the treatment of subfertility is controversial. Whilst it may result in improved semen parameters, this may not necessarily be reflected in improved pregnancy rates. The European Association of Urology (EAU) guidelines currently recommend the treatment of men with a clinical varicocele, oligozoospermia, and otherwise unexplained infertility in the couple, although it accepts that the evidence for this is weak.

The mainstay of treatment is varicocele embolization. Success rates are around 85%. Surgical treatments involve ligation of the testicular veins via a sub inguinal (Marmar), inguinal (Ivanissevich), or laparoscopic approach. Success rates of 95% have been quoted. Whichever treatment modality is used, discharging the patient on the day of the procedure is feasible.

Testicular Cancer + Radical Inguinal Orchidectomy

Testicular cancer accounts for 5% of all urological cancers and is the commonest solid cancer in men between the ages of 20–45 years. The incidence is increasing with a peak in the third and fourth decades. Owing to its sensitivity to platinum-based chemotherapy regimens, in general, the prognosis is excellent.

Most patients will present to the general urology clinic having detected a lump in the testes. This is usually otherwise asymptomatic although pain can be present in approximately 5% of cases. It is essential that these patients are seen urgently with a diagnosis confirmed on ultrasound and tumour markers sent (alpha fetoprotein, beta-human chorionic gonadotropin (βhCG), and lactate dehydrogenase (LDH)). Prior to surgery, patients should also be offered semen preservation. Computerized tomography (CT) for staging (abdomen, pelvis ± chest) is also arranged.

Radical inguinal orchidectomy is the primary treatment option in almost all patients (except those who present with high volume metastatic disease). This may be performed in conjunction with insertion of a testicular prosthesis and contralateral testicular biopsy.

The procedure is performed through a groin incision approximately 2 cm above and parallel to the inguinal ligament. The external oblique aponeurosis is identified (along with the ilio-inguinal nerve just below it) and incised to expose the cord. Early clamping of the cord adjacent to the internal ring is performed. The testicle is then delivered and the gubernaculum divided. The cord is cut between two clamps and ligated with heavy sutures. A non-absorbable suture may be used to aid identification during any future lymph node dissection. Haemostasis and vascular pedicle control are essential because a bleeding, retracted cord can be difficult to control. A prosthesis, if requested, is then inserted and closure performed with generous local anaesthetic infiltration of the wound. The majority of patients (who are usually young and with few co-morbidities) will be discharged with dressings the same day.

Phimosis and Circumcision

Tightness of the foreskin, which cannot be retracted behind the glans penis, affects both adults and children. Physiological phimosis present at birth usually resolves such that less than 1% of 17-year-old males have a persistent phimosis. The indications for circumcision in the paediatric population is, therefore, reserved for pathological phimosis resulting in recurrent balanitis, recurrent urinary tract infections (UTIs) or the presence of balanitis xerotica obliterans (BXO).

In the adult male, recurrent balanitis or BXO can result in pathological phimosis. Mild phimosis may be asymptomatic. Depending on the age of the patient and severity of the phimosis, the patient may develop symptoms of bleeding, splitting, difficulty with sexual intercourse and voiding problems. A tight phimosis may also result in a paraphimosis in which the foreskin becomes stuck behind the glans and cannot be replaced. This requires urgent attention to prevent glans necrosis developing.

Phimosis may respond to topical steroids but these have often been tried in the primary care setting before the patient is referred to the urology clinic. Preputioplasty is an alternative to a full circumcision in cases of a mild phimosis.

There are multiple ways to perform a circumcision. Whichever technique is used, it is imperative the (often young) patient has a full understanding of the procedure and its associated complications, especially decreased glans sensitivity and poor cosmesis. General principles for circumcision are the use of a penile block, bipolar diathermy, and meticulous haemostasis (particularly with regard to the frenular artery). The patient can be safely discharged on the day of surgery with dressings and wound care advice.

Peyronie's Disease and Penile Straightening Surgery

Peyronie's disease affects up to 7% of men. It is characterised by penile deviation due to fibrous plaque formation on the tunica albuginea. Penile deviation is a consequence of the inability of corpora cavernosum underlying the plaque to lengthen on erection in relation to the rest of the penis. The exact aetiology of the condition is unknown although it is thought to be an inflammatory connective tissue disorder related to repeated micro-trauma. It is characterised by an acute (active) and a chronic (stable) phase. It is important that any surgical correction is deferred until the chronic phase of the disease, once stabilisation of the plaque has occurred.

Most patients will present with penile deviation, a palpable lump (plaque) and/or pain on erection. It is essential to obtain a history regarding any co-existing or new erectile dysfunction. It is useful to ask patients to bring a photo with them to the clinic to assess the degree of deviation and progress over time.

Patients can be managed conservatively, medically, or surgically. There is limited evidence of the efficacy of medical treatments such as Vitamin E, tamoxifen, or POTABA.

The two most commonly used surgical procedures to treat Peyronie's disease are Nesbitt's and Lue's procedures. Nesbitt's procedure aims to correct the deformity by incising an ellipse of tunica albuginea on the unaffected side. It is generally indicated when the degree of deviation is <60%. In Lue's procedure, an incision on the plaque on the affected side is performed with insertion of a graft. Patients must be informed of the risks of post-operative erectile dysfunction and loss of erect penile length. In patients who present with Peyronie's disease and moderate to severe erectile dysfunction, insertion of a penile prosthesis may be offered.

Whilst these procedures are increasingly being performed in specialist centres, all may be feasibly carried out as a day-case.

Vasectomy

Vasectomies are performed as a form of male contraception. In the UK currently, many vasectomies are being carried out in the primary care setting. Often, patients requesting vasectomies are seen in the urology clinic only if it is thought not to be straightforward e.g. in the context of previous scrotal surgery or a patient's request for general anaesthesia. Even so, a vasectomy performed in hospital is still ideally suited to be performed as a day case.

The procedure can be performed under either local or general anaesthetic. Various techniques are described and either a single or two incisions used. General principles of technique are to isolate the vas deferens between thumb and forefingers, incise the skin over the vas, then lift the vas away from the scrotum by incising the sheath surrounding it. A 1–2 cm segment of vas is then excised and the ends are occluded. This can be achieved by diathermy, clips, and suture ligation with or without a fascial interposition.

It is essential that men requesting a vasectomy have a full understanding of the procedure, risks, and alternatives. The consent process must highlight that the procedure should be considered irreversible, the risks of primary and secondary failure, bleeding, infection, chronic pain, and the need for contraception until either a semen analysis shows no sperm after at least 12 weeks and 20 ejaculations or special clearance has been given by a doctor.

Further Reading

BMJ Best Practice - Hydrocele (2020). https://bestpractice.bmj.com/topics/en-gb/1104.

Hancock, P., Woodward, B.J., Muneer, A. et al. (2016). 2016 laboratory guidelines for post vasectomy semen analysis. *J. Clin. Path.* 69: 655–660.

Laguna MP, Albers P, Algaba F et al. (2019). EAU Guidelines on testicular cancer. http://uroweb.org/guideline/testicular-cancer.

Riddick, A. (1998). Testicular lumps in general practice. *Practitioner* 242 (1590): 627–630.

13

Ambulatory Management of Renal Stone Disease
Aakash Pai

Epidemiology

Urinary stones are the third most common affliction of the urinary tract, super-seded only by infection and prostatic pathologies. The incidence of calculi is increasing, with prevalence rates in countries such as the United States, Sweden, and the UK more than 9%. Men have an increased risk of urolithiasis compared to women; however, this difference in incidence is reducing. Stones can occur in all ages; however, the peak age is approximately 45. The risk of stone formation has shown correlation with body mass index and with certain diseases including diabetes mellitus and cardiovascular disease.

Aetiology

Urinary stones have been affecting humans, and dogs, for civilisations. Despite this, much of the aetiology of urolithiasis is unknown. Stone formation comprises a complex cascade. Urine becomes supersaturated with stone forming salts, with a resultant precipitation out of solution, forming crystals or nuclei. These crystals can be retained within the kidney at anchoring sites that promote growth and aggression and resultant stone formation.

Stone formation is related to supersaturation of urine. The *solubility product* is the concentration product a solution reaches where no further added salt crystals will dissolve. Below the solubility product, urine is *undersaturated* and crystals do not form. Above the solubility product, crystals should form, but don't because of inhibitors in urine. Above a certain concentration, inhibitors become ineffective, urine is *supersaturated,* and the concentration of solute at which this is reached

Ambulatory Urology and Urogynaecology, First Edition. Edited by Abhay Rane and Ajay Rane.

(crystallisation starts) is the *formation product*. Urine is *metastable* between the solubility product and formation product.

Supersaturation explains the formation of crystals in static solutions, but it cannot explain crystal formation in urine as it traverses through the nephron. Crystals form (nucleation) and if they aggregate together, they may retain in the lumen and grow (*free particle theory*). Alternatively, they may attach to damaged tubular surfaces (*fixed particle theory*).

Types of Stones

Non-infection stones

Calcium oxalate

Calcium phosphate

Uric acid

Infection stones

Magnesium ammonium phosphate

Carbonate apatite

Ammonium urate

Genetic causes

Cystine

Xanthine

2,8-Dihydroxyadenine

Drug stones

Risk Factors

Diseases associated with stone formation

Hyperparathyroidism

Metabolic syndrome

Nephrocalcinosis

Polycystic kidney disease

Gastrointestinal diseases and bariatric surgery

Sarcoidosis

Spinal cord injury

Genetically determined stone formation

Cystinuria

Primary hyperoxaluria

Renal tubular acidosis type I

Drug-induced stone formation, e.g., antiretroviral stones (Indinavir)

Anatomical abnormalities associated with stone formation

Medullary sponge kidney (tubular ectasia)

Pelviureteric obstruction

Calyceal diverticulae

Environmental factors

High temperature

Symptoms

Ureteric stones commonly present with sudden onset severe flank pain. The pain is commonly colicky (waves of increasing severity followed by reduced severity pain) and may radiate from the loin to the groin.

Signs

Fifty percent of loin pain is non-urological in nature and therefore careful inspection of the patient is necessary. Patients with ureteric colic usually twist and roll, trying to find a comfortable position. Conversely, patients suffering from conditions that cause peritonitis classically lie completely still. It is important to ensure that the patient is afebrile.

Investigation

It is imperative to perform a pregnancy test in any premenopausal female. Many patients with ureteric colic have non-visible haematuria, however 10–30% have no blood in their urine. Computed tomography of kidneys, ureters, and bladder (CT KUB) is the gold standard diagnostic test for presumed ureteric colic with a sensitivity of 99%. Blood tests including renal function should be taken.

Emergency Management of the Infected Obstructed System

The septic patient with an obstructed system is a urological emergency. Immediate intravenous fluid resuscitation, urine and blood cultures, intravenous antibiotics, and emergency decompression should be organised. Definitive stone management should be delayed until after the sepsis has resolved. The oft quoted randomised controlled trial by Pearle et al. (1998), showed that both stent and nephrostomy were equally effective in decompression of 42 patients with an infected obstructed system. The method of decompression is therefore at the discretion of the urologist, depending upon patient, stone, and logistical considerations.

Treatment

Conservative

Obstructing ureteric stones with manageable levels of pain, no signs of infection and the absence of marked renal failure can be considered for conservative management and discharge home. The success of the conservative management of ureteric colic is dependant primarily on stone size and location. Expectant management is usually reserved for stones less than 10 mm, with distal ureteric stones less than 5 mm the most likely to pass. Consideration should be given to the fact that the pelvic brim and vesico-ureteric junction are smaller in calibre than the upper ureter and stones found to be lodged in the upper ureter on imaging are therefore less likely to pass spontaneously.

Medical expulsive therapy (MET) with an alpha-blocker medication is contentious; whilst it is a theoretically sound treatment, large scale randomised controlled trials have not reliably confirmed efficacy and many surgeons are now abandoning this treatment.

Patients should be discharged home with adequate analgesia (a non-steroidal anti-inflammatory and an opioid) and given clear instructions to return to hospital in the event of worsened pain or onset of any kind of fever or malaise.

Ideally, patients should be followed up in an outpatient clinic after two weeks for repeat imaging on the day with either ultrasound or plain x-ray to confirm stone progress or passage. This allows adequate time to arrange alternative ambulatory therapy for cases in which successful stone passage appears unlikely, before irreversible renal damage begins to occur.

Extracorporeal Shock Wave Lithotripsy

Extracorporeal shock wave lithotripsy (ESWL) is a valuable modality for the ambulatory treatment of renal and lower ureteric stones. Relatively compact 'mobile' ESWL machines can be quickly set up in any clinical of adequate size with a suitable power source. Consideration may need to be given to adequate shielding if x-rays are to be used for stone visualisation, and contingency plans must be drawn up for emergency care in the exceptionally rare events of a reaction to medication, bleeding, or cardiac arrythmia developing due to shock waves. Most units performing ESWL will use NSAID medication as analgesia, but small doses of midazolam or pethidine are also commonly in use to ensure a comfortable treatment that is compatible with an ambulatory approach.

As with all stone management, the suitability for, and success of, ESWL is dependent on stone factors (size, location, Hounsfield units), patient factors (preference, obesity, anticoagulation, and severe hypertension) and anatomical factors (calyceal anatomy). Lower ureteric stones can be considered for ESWL treatment; however, generally ESWL is used more often for stones within the collecting system. ESWL is not preferred for stones >10 mm, lower pole location, stones within calyceal diverticulae, patients with pelviureteric juncture (PUJ) obstruction and hard calcium monohydrate calculi.

Uretero-renoscopy

Small-calibre deflecting ureteroscopes coupled with the development of stone baskets and high-power Holmium: YAG (yttrium aluminium garnet) lasers mean that the popularity and indications for uretero renoscopy have increased. The advent of single-use flexible ureteroscopes (such as the Pusen U-Scope) has introduced reliable, high-fidelity visuals for every case and, in some cases, superior manoeuvrability and deflection as compared 're-usable' flexible cystoscopes. In the majority of cases, the entire collecting system can be accessed by these modern scopes, thus maximising chances of successfully rendering a patient 'stone free' with a single ambulatory visit.

Holmium laser is highly absorbed by water and has a very small penetration depth of approximately 0.4 mm, making it a safe option for stone fragmentation during ureteroscopy. Success rates are generally higher than for ESWL. Ureteroscopy is performed under general anaesthesia in most units, but several authors have reported excellent experiences performing the procedure under local anaesthesia. Even with general anaesthesia and even if neuromuscular blockage is required to minimise respiratory movement for collecting system stones, same-day discharge is still easily achieved as long as the patient recovers from surgery with sufficient analgesia. As with other treatment modalities, NSAIDS and opioids are mainstays of pain control.

Traditionally stones >2 cm are treated with percutaneous nephrolithotomy (PCNL), however larger stones are now being tackled via the ureteroscope, although evidence of the efficacy of this approach is still evolving.

PCNL

Stones greater than 2 cm, inaccessible stones and those that have failed other modalities are usually treated with percutaneous nephrolithonomy (PCNL). PCNL has the highest stone free rates out of all modalities for renal calculi. Direct collecting system puncture and stone fragmentation is technically a more invasive procedure than ureteroscopy; however, the concept of a 'tubeless' PCNL (where no nephrostomy is left in place after the procedure) allowed the first possibility of the procedure being compatible with same-day discharge. The last decade has also seen the use of smaller tract sizes for PCNL; mini-PCNL employs tract sizes at 14–20 Fr, ultra-mini is 11–13 Fr and micro-PCNL is 4.85 Fr. This 'miniaturisation' has allowed an ever-increasing proportion or larger stones to be managed as ambulatory surgery. Whilst smaller tracts are associated with improved length of stay and reduced morbidity, but there is a potential for reduced stone clearance.

ESWL's lack of anaesthesia, the popularity of miniaturised PCNL tracts, and the increased capability of ureteroscopes mean that there is an increasing overlap between the indications for the respective modalities. The decision for the intervention of choice is hence individualised; based upon patient and clinician preference.

Long-Term Management and Prevention

Serum calcium should be checked in all stone patients. Stones should be sent for analysis of their composition. 24-hour urine analysis should be considered for those patients who are at high risk (e.g., young adult and paediatric patients, recurrent high-volume stone formers).

Long-term prevention of renal calculi centres around ensuring a high fluid intake (at least 2.5 l water a day). In addition, carbonated drinks should be avoided, and the addition of fresh lemon juice to drinking water can be protective. Adults should limit their salt intake (no more than 6 g a day). Calcium intake should not be restricted. A reduced intake of meat and maintaining a healthy body mass index (BMI) are also advisable.

Urinary alkalinisation with potassium citrate should be considered for patients with recurrent stones that are predominantly composed of calcium oxalate. Thiazide diuretics are an option in patients with recurrent calcium oxalate stones and hypercalciuria.

Further Reading

Lingeman, J.E., Siegel, Y.I., Steele, B. et al. (1994). Management of lower pole nephrolithiasis: a critical analysis. *J. Urol.* 151: 663–667.

Pearle, M.S., Lingeman, J.E., Leveillee, R. et al. (2015). Prospective, randomized trial comparing shock wave lithotripsy and ureteroscopy for lower pole calculi 1 cm or less. *J. Urol.* 173 (6): 2005–2009.

Pearle, M.S., Pierce, H.L., Miller, G.L. et al. (1998 Oct). Optimal method of urgent decompression of the collecting system for obstruction and infection due to ureteral calculi. *J Urol.* 160 (4): 1260–1264.

Turk, C., Petrik, A., Sarica, K. et al. (2016). EAU guidelines on diagnosis and conservative management of urolithiasis. *Eur. Urol.* 69 (3): 468–474.

14

The Management of Recurrent Urinary Tract Infections

Jordan Durrant

Urinary tract infections are a common issue in the urology outpatient clinic and effective management is key in preventing future hospitalisation and inpatient emergency admission. Unfortunately, it is not uncommon for the information received in a referral for a patient with recurrent urinary tract infections (rUTI) to be less than is required to make a full assessment of the patient. Therefore, history taking is paramount in determining the exact cause of the patient's complaints and formulating a treatment strategy.

The majority of patients will be referred to your clinic with complaints of **cystitis** – inflammation of the urothelium and bladder, presumed to be due to infection and invasion of bacteria. It is this scenario that is discussed in this chapter.

History

In addition to a more generalised past medical history that makes note of conditions that may contribute to rUTI (diabetes, menopause, immunosuppression, etc.), it is important to take a full history of the patient's complaints regarding their cystitis symptoms. A note should be made of symptoms and signs that support the diagnosis of rUTI:

- Recurrent episodes of frequency and urgency/irritative voiding symptoms
- Associated supra-pubic discomfort/pain
- Associated dysuria
- Offensive and/or purulent urine
- General malaise, fever, and associated systemic symptoms
- A predictable and recognised trigger for an episode (intercourse, dehydration, etc.)

Ambulatory Urology and Urogynaecology, First Edition. Edited by Abhay Rane and Ajay Rane.
© 2021 John Wiley & Sons Ltd. Published 2021 by John Wiley & Sons Ltd.

- Positive/confirmatory mid-stream urine (MSU) culture results
- Response to antibiotic therapy

In the absence of supporting evidence from the patient history, consideration should be given to other possible diagnoses. For example, irritative voiding symptoms with recurrent bouts of visible haematuria and bacterial growth on MSU may be a presentation of a bladder tumour (around half of bladder tumours are colonised by bacteria). Alternatively, in the absence of positive microbiology, bouts of irritative voiding symptoms with supra-pubic pain relieved by voiding is indicative of Bladder Pain Syndrome.

Lastly, a brief history of any lower urinary tract symptoms (LUTS) at other times should be sought.

If a true diagnosis of rUTI is suspected, potential risk factors should be identified as part of history taking (see below).

Definitions

Recurrent urinary tract infection is generally accepted to mean more than two infections in a six-month period, or more than three episodes in a year.

Significant bacteriuria was originally defined by Kass as $>10^5$ cfu/ml. Most hospital laboratories still adhere to this 'cut-off.' However, it is important to be aware that in many patients with frequent proven infections some apparently 'negative' MSU samples (which indicate pyuria), may have growth of $<10^5$ cfu/ml and, in fact, there may be meaningful bacteriuria. Indeed, the European Urology Association now recognises $>10^3$ cfu/ml as significant.

Re-Infection is the development of a further infection several months after a previous episode, whereas bacterial persistence can result in more frequent episodes of infection and is likely frequently underestimated as a cause for many presentations of rUTI.

Risk Factors and Patient Discussion

A great deal of 'common sense' knowledge regarding potential risk factors for development of rUTI is backed by good evidence. Certainly, no urologist would argue that a male with a chronic urinary retention of 1 litre is at risk of infection, but on a lesser scale there is no evidence to support the idea that a female with a post-void residual of 150 ml is at any greater risk of developing infection than a female with a 25 ml residual.

Personal Hygiene

Common advice to females regarding avoidance of bubble-baths and vaginal douching and ensuring passage of urine after coitus have also not been proven to lower the risk of UTI, even if the advice is logical.

Genetics

Some risk factors are not modifiable, but may be of interest to patients with rUTI. There is compelling evidence of a genetic predisposition to rUTI in some patients. A large case control study has shown that in women, having a mother with rUTI was a risk factor for developing the condition. The P1 blood group phenotype also confers risk.

Fluid Intake

Inadequate fluid intake is associated with rUTI risk. It has been shown that people who restrict their fluid intake during working hours for convenience have a more than twofold increase in UTI risk as compared to controls.

Intercourse

The relationship between coitus and episodes of UTI is controversial. No reliable link between intercourse and UTI is demonstrated in the literature. Some literature demonstrates a direct correlation, whereas other researchers have found no association between intercourse frequency and positive urine cultures. Anecdotally, this appears to be born out in the outpatient clinic, where some women report no association, whilst others report a predictable association (discussed further later). There is compelling evidence, however, that intercourse with condom or spermicide usage raises the risk of infection. No evidence exists though to support the common advice for women to pass urine post-coitus, to prevent UTI.

Menopause

Loss of oestrogens during menopause results in a rise in vaginal pH. Low pH (below 4.5) virtually inhibits vaginal colonisation. Post-menopausal females with rUTI can benefit from topical oestrogens because it lowers pH and bacterial colonisation. Indeed, at lower pH levels, there is increased growth of lactobacillus, which itself also serves to inhibit unwanted colonisation.

Biofilms and QIRs

In animal studies it has been demonstrated that uropathogenic *Escherichia coli* forms intra-cellular niches within urothelial facet cells. These 'quiescent intracellular reservoirs' (QIRs) persist following resolution of an infection and are highly likely to play in role in relapsing infections. It should be born in mind that the urothelium has a long 'turnover time' of approximately 200 days. This potentially means that a facet cell containing bacteria may persist for six months.

In recent years, our understanding of the role of biofilms in rUTI has increased. Biofilms are sessile bacterial communities attached to a substrate and each other, embedded within extracellular polymeric substances that they have produced. These organisms exhibit altered phenotypes and growth patterns that confer increased resistance to their elimination.

Further Advice to the Patient

As discussed earlier, improving fluid intake appears to be a useful measure in lowering the risk of rUTI episodes. Much is made of the advice to void after intercourse, avoid bubble-baths and avoid certain underwear types, however, this advice is not backed by evidence.

Cranberry juice and cranberry extract are often touted as a natural remedy for rUTI. The usefulness of this intervention has been examined twice in Cochrane reviews, and it was reported that cranberry usage has no statistically significant effect of UTI frequency.

Another 'natural' remedy that appeals to patients is the use of probiotics. As discussed earlier, lactobacilli cell walls have an inhibitory effect on coliform colonisation. The use of both oral ingestion of lactobacilli preparations and vaginal use of probiotics and lactobacilli was examined in a Cochrane review, there was no strong evidence to support recommending it to patients.

Investigation

In the outpatient clinic, urine dipstick testing is an essential tool for routine investigation. If available, uroflowmetry and post-micturition residual volume measurement may be indicated in patients who give a history suggestive of associated LUTS.

Generally, further investigation will have a low diagnostic yield. However, renal tract ultrasound may reveal anatomical abnormalities in a small proportion of females with recurrent and difficult to treat infections.

A pattern of haematuria or persistent haematuria should raise concerns of underlying bladder malignancy and be urgently investigated by cystoscopy.

The presence of proteus or repeated culture of other urea-splitting organisms should prompt suspicion of nephrolithiasis.

Management Strategies

Recurrent urinary tract infection has the potential to be a distressing problem for the patient and one that is difficult to manage for the clinician. A number of evidence-based approaches to the issue exist.

Continuous Antimicrobials

Unsurprisingly, antibiotic usage is a highly effective way of managing the issue. There is evidence across multiple studies that continuous low-dose prophylaxis reduces the risk of a confirmed UTI by 80%. Multiple studies have shown this risk reduction effect persisting for a period after discontinuation of antibiotics, giving credence to the theory of biofilms in intracellular reservoirs.

From a practical viewpoint, a period of low-dose prophylaxis is likely to be one of the first measures recommended for patients with difficult to treat rUTI. Choice of antibiotic agent should be informed by evidence from MSU cultures and local microbiology policies. Nitrofurantoin is likely the most evidenced antimicrobial, but is not suitable for indefinite usage.

There is no strong evidence to make recommendations on length of low-dose prophylaxis treatment. Many trials have been of 6-months duration, there is limited evidence that 12-month courses are associated with a longer period of risk-reduction following discontinuation. The decision ultimately is at the clinician's discretion. However, modern understanding of QIRs and biofilms has seen a trend towards longer, rather than shorter, periods of low-dose prophylaxis.

Self-Directed Prophylaxis

Numerous researchers have examined the effectiveness and ability of patients to direct their own antibiotic usage. This is potentially a treatment strategy for less severe of recurrent infections or suitable for management of infections following cessation of continuous prophylaxis. Although contentious (see above), women who report an association between intercourse and UTI experience a significant reduction in UTI episodes when using self-directed antibiotics post-coitally. Furthermore, it has been demonstrated that women reliably identify their own bacteriuria based on symptoms alone, allowing self-directed treatment to be appropriately instigated after the onset of symptoms.

D-Mannose

D-Mannose is widely available in health shops and may be of use in patients with recurrent coliform cystitis. Ingested D-Mannose is excreted in urine and binds to Type I Pili on uropathogenic *E. coli*, preventing subsequent adhesion to mannosylated residues on the bladder surface. In a small randomised controlled trial, D-Mannose was found to significantly reduce risk of UTI episode and was comparable to nitrofurantoin. In daily practice, most clinicians who advise D-Mannose find it to be useful for some patients but not for others.

Methenamine Hippurate

This oral preparation has long been known to produce excretion of formaldehyde in the urine, which can serve to sterilise the urine. Multiple small studies have demonstrated its ability to reduce the incidence of infection, albeit less effectively than nitrofurantoin. It is a key option for on-going prophylaxis for patients who continue to suffer infections after initial treatment. A small proportion of patients will experience gastrointestinal upset as a side effect.

Vaccines

A number of different vaccine preparations are commercially available for the management of rUTI. These vaccines frequently come in the form of vaginal suppositories containing a mixture of heat-killed bacterial strains. Whilst their exact mechanism of action remains unproven, it has been demonstrated that administration of such vaccines increases levels of IgA and IgG at the introitus.

An oral preparation containing 18 heat-killed serotypes has been demonstrated to reduce relative risk of UTI recurrence by almost 40%.

GAG Layer Treatments

The glycosaminoglycan (GAG) layer forms a mucous barrier over the superficial facet cells in the bladder. Theoretically, deficiency or poor differentiation of this layer allows bacteria to adhere more easily and penetrate facet cells and form biofilms.

Existing treatments for replenishing and reinforcing the GAG layer have been proposed as a management for rUTI. Multiple studies have shown that sodium hyaluronate containing bladder instillations, when given in an induction and monthly maintenance schedule, reduce UTI rate by approximately 70–80%, Unfortunately, this is an expensive and time-consuming treatment modality. However, the advent of preparations designed for self-administration increase the scope for use of these treatments in the future.

Further Reading

Albert, X., Huertas, I., Inmaculado, P. et al. (2004). Antibiotics for preventing recurrent urinary tract infection in non-pregnant women. *Cochrane Database of Systematic Reviews* 3: CD001209.

Lee, B.S., Bhuta, T., Simpson, J.M. et al. (2012). Methenamine hippurate for preventing urinary tract infections. *Cochrane Database of Systematic Reviews* 10: CD003265.

Mysorekar, I.U. and Hultgren, S.J. (2006). Mechanisms of uropathogenic Escherichia Coli persistence and eradication from the urinary tract. *Proceedings of the National Academy of Sciences of the United States of America* 103 (38): 14170–14175.

15

An Ambulatory Approach to Benign Prostatic Obstruction

Tharani Mahesan

Perhaps the most common presentation to a urology clinic is the male patient with lower urinary tract symptoms (LUTS). Patients may present to a general urology clinic, via a 'raised prostate specific antigen (PSA) clinic' or as a result of a failed trial without catheter (TWOC). Many urology units are now striving to offer a merged 'one-stop' clinic for all such conditions, and LUTS is a condition that lends itself well to the ethos of ambulatory care. In a well-organised service, it should be possible to offer all necessary investigations and assessments in order to reach a diagnosis and plan treatment for the male LUTS patient.

Lower urinary tract symptoms may be divided into storage and voiding symptoms. This differentiation is made on patient history and dictates appropriate investigation. In patients with solely storage symptoms (urgency of urination, frequency, and nocturia), diagnoses such as infection, overactive bladder (OAB) syndrome, or detrusor overactivity (DO) should be considered. Patients with voiding symptoms (hesitancy, poor flow, intermittency, double voiding) and those with mixed voiding and storage symptoms are more likely to have bladder outflow obstruction as the underlying cause.

Bladder outflow obstruction must be considered in men presenting with urinary tract infection, orchitis, acute urinary retention, bladder stones, and also those with high post-void residual volumes in the bladder and indications of chronic urinary retention.

Bladder outflow obstruction is, to a degree, considered synonymous with benign prostatic obstruction (BPO) and benign prostatic hyperplasia (BPH). Indeed, 50% of men have BPH by the age of 60. However, other causes of obstruction are not infrequent and should be excluded. Other diagnoses to consider should include urethral stricture disease, bladder neck stenosis, detrusor failure, and obstruction due to prostate cancer or urothelial cancer.

Ambulatory Urology and Urogynaecology, First Edition. Edited by Abhay Rane and Ajay Rane.
© 2021 John Wiley & Sons Ltd. Published 2021 by John Wiley & Sons Ltd.

Table 15.1 Distinguishing between differential diagnoses.

Alternative diagnosis to BPO as a cause of LUTS	Investigations
Bladder neck stenosis	Should be considered in men who have undergone previous transurethral resection of the prostate (TURP) or radical prostatectomy.
	Can be diagnosed on flexible cystoscopy.
Urethral stricture	Very poor Qmax
	Classic appearance of flat flow rate on uroflowmetry
	Should be considered in men with previous history of stricture, radiotherapy or trauma but can be present without.
	Can be diagnosed on flexible cystoscopy.
Prostate cancer	Should be considered as a potential diagnosis in all men >50 years of age.
	Digital rectal exam (DRE) may demonstrate nodules, asymmetry or a firm prostate.
	Raised PSA (>3.5 ng/ml).
	Check for family history.
	Investigate further with magnetic resonance imaging (MRI) and consideration of biopsy.
'Bladder failure' aka detrusor underactivity (DU)	Should be considered in men re-presenting after prior bladder outlet obstruction (BOO) surgery.
	Urodynamic testing will demonstrate low voiding pressure, intermittent flow and incomplete bladder emptying. A calculated Bladder Contractility Index <100 is considered diagnostic.

Several tools can be utilised in distinguishing between these aetiologies, and the findings of such investigations are summarised in Table 15.1.

Further Assessment and Investigations

History

Crucial in any urology clinic is the history from the patient. It is important to establish the nature, duration, and bother of his LUTS. One should attempt to elicit which aspect of his LUTS he finds most bothersome, although other tools will also help to elucidate that.

Table 15.2 Urine dipstick testing interpretation.

Outcome of urine dipstick analysis	Action
Blood	Microscopic haematuria can indicate the presence of a urothelial cancer.
	Patients with this require investigation with a flexible cystoscopy and upper tract imaging. Urine cytology can also be offered.
Glucose	This may indicate a diagnosis of diabetes mellitus and predispose to symptoms such as frequency and nocturia. The patient's regular doctor may need to investigate this further prior to urological intervention.
Leucocytes +/− nitrite	If this finding is associated with symptoms of dysuria and irritative LUTS may be associated urinary tract infection. In such instances a mid-stream urine sample should be sent for culture and antibiotics commenced.

The patient's regular doctor may have commenced medications and it is important to establish what those are. Enquire about past medical history as well as associated medications because several widely used medications are known to have urological consequences despite being prescribed for non-urological problems (e.g., alpha-blocker medication maybe prescribed for blood pressure control and amitriptyline is associated with urinary retention).

It must be established whether any previous urological surgery has been undertaken and consideration should be given to prostate cancer if there is a significant family history. It is important to identify any 'red-flag' symptoms such as visible haematuria, weight loss, or anorexia.

Basic investigations should include urine dipstick testing (see Table 15.2), serum PSA, and urea and electrolytes testing to assess renal function.

Perhaps most important is to elicit the patient's expectations around the referral. Many are concerned about the risk of prostate cancer and steps should be taken to prove the absence of such disease in order to offer reassurance.

Urine Dipstick Testing

A urine dip is a non-invasive, easily available bedside test that can be used to identify other causes of LUTS.

Prostate Examination and PSA

An irregular prostate on digital rectal exam (DRE) may be an indication of prostate cancer and requires prompt investigation with a PSA and MRI in order to exclude a diagnosis of prostate cancer. A prostate exam also provides clinicians with an idea of prostate size. This can be useful later in determining choice of surgical intervention.

Clinicians should remember that PSA can be artificially elevated in chronic retention and urinary tract infection. Invasive investigations such as flexible cystoscopy can produce appreciable but transient PSA elevations for up to six weeks afterwards.

Uroflowmetry

Uroflowmetry allows the clinician a non-invasive assessment or urinary flow dynamics. Key data include voided volume, maximum flow speed (Qmax), and voiding time. An ultrasound is routinely performed after a flow test to establish the volume of urine remaining in the bladder, also known as a post-void residual (PVR).

Modern urology units most commonly employ pressure transducers (electronic weight scales) to measure the volume of urine voided by the patient and to calculate the speed at which that weight change has occurred. This rate of change is represented on a 'flow chart' diagram. Flow speed (ml/s) is plotted on the x-axis, with voiding time on the y-axis. A normal flow pattern will appear as bell-curve, skewed slightly along the y-axis. The maximum peak (Q-Max) of the curve should reach around 25 ml/s.

Results should be interpreted with caution as flow rates do not necessarily differentiate between causes of obstructions and the risk of artefact secondary to a wandering flow is high. (See Table 15.3.) Uroflowmetry where the voided flow is less than 150 ml is not considered diagnostically useful.

Urodynamic Studies

Urodynamic studies are employed in the assessment of suspected BPO to confirm or refute the presence of obstruction. It should be considered in men with equivocal flow rates, those who are young and wishing to avoid inappropriate surgical intervention or very elderly patients for whom surgery poses increased risk. Patients with a potential neurogenic component to their symptoms (e.g., CVA or Parkinson's disease) and patient's representing with refractory symptoms following surgery should also be strongly considered for investigation.

Modern Urodynamics equipment offers automated calculation of the likelihood of obstructed flow using the Abrams Griffiths nomogram or an equivalent. Close

Table 15.3   Interpretation of uroflowmetry results.

Flow rate finding	Suggested Diagnosis
Flat flow rate with long voiding time and poor Qmax	Stricture
Flow rate rises quickly to Qmax and is then maintained	Normal
Poor flow rate, with slow rise to peak, failure to maintain and intermittency	Obstructed
Qmax <10 ml/s	Likelihood of obstruction is 90%
Qmax 10–14 ml/s	Likelihood of obstruction is 67%
Qmax >15 ml/s	Likelihood of obstruction is 30%

scrutiny of results (i.e. the Pdet Qmax) is still required to ensure that the computer software has correctly identified the voiding phase of the study and has based the calculation on detrusor pressures during this period.

Flexible Cystoscopy

Discussed further in Chapter 18, Urothelial Bladder Cancer, a flexible cystoscopy can provide further evaluation of the lower urinary tract. It can be used to quickly confirm the presence of urethral stricture disease and to assess prostate shape and anatomy (which may impact choice of surgical intervention). It can also identify features of high filling pressure within the bladder, such as diverticulae and trabeculation. Cystoscopy cannot identify obstruction, but the finding of a large or occlusive prostate may lead one to suspect it.

Ultrasound and Post Void Residual Volume Measurement

In an ambulatory urology service, an ultrasound scanner (with a moderate degree of training) can be used to add vital detail to the assessment of a patient with benign prostate obstruction (BPO).

Ultrasound allows the clinician to make rapid assessments of urine volume within the bladder and prostate volume and size (more accurately if a trans-rectal probe is used) and with training; hydronephrosis and upper urinary tract dilatation may be identified in patients with high pressure chronic retention – indicating a potential need for inpatient admission following catheterisation.

Post-void residual volume measurements of up to 300 ml are generally considered acceptable, if high. Residual volumes in the range of 150–300 mls may imply an element of BPO. Post-void residuals over 300 ml are indicative of chronic urinary retention. More than 1000 ml within the bladder is considered a potential indicator of high-pressure retention (whether an 'acute on chronic' retention or simply chronic). These patients are at risk of developing a post-obstructive diuresis following catheterisation and should be considered for inpatient admission and observation, especially when renal function is deranged.

International Prostate Symptom Score

The International Prostate Symptom Score (IPSS) is a short, validated patient questionnaire that allows rapid assessment of patient symptoms, using a seven-question scoring system. Scores range between 0 and 35. An eighth, separate question relates to the impact of these symptoms on the patient's quality of life. Scores of 0–7 correlate with mild symptoms and scores of 20–35 indicate severe symptoms.

An IPSS is useful in guiding treatment decisions (lifestyle advice alone is unlikely to prove useful with an IPSS of 25), establishing the extent of bother, and assisting with the process of differentiating between storage and voiding symptoms.

Medical Management

All discussions of management should begin with appropriate lifestyle modification advice. Common guidance includes avoiding fluids before bedtime for those with nocturia, and avoiding caffeine for those with irritative storage symptoms.

First line medication for patients with bladder outflow obstruction secondary to benign prostatic hyperplasia (BPH) should be an α-blocker medication, such as Tamsulosin. This selective α1-receptor antagonist relaxes smooth muscle in the bladder neck and prostate to reduce bladder outflow resistance. Patients should be cautioned on the risk of postural hypotension as well as the likelihood of retrograde ejaculation and floppy iris syndrome. Tamsulosin can take up to 3 days to take effect and 14 days for maximum effect.

In severely symptomatic cases of BPO or cases refractory to α-blocker treatment, a 5 α-reductase inhibitor such Finasteride or Dutasteride can be offered in combination with Tamsulosin. These medications limit the bio-active testosterone that drives prostatic hypertrophy. Trials such as medical therapy of prostatic symptoms (MTOPS) and combination of Avodart (dutasteride) and Tamsulosin (combAT) have consistently demonstrated the superior benefit of dual-agent therapy over single therapy, either in terms of reduction in progression of symptoms or reduction of symptoms.

Patients who cannot tolerate Tamsulosin can be prescribed Finasteride alone. Finasteride can take up to six months for significant improvements to become apparent and is associated with side effects including sexual dysfunction such as impotence, loss of libido, and erectile dysfunction in around 5% of patients.

Surgical Management

For men in whom medical management is inadequate, unsuccessful, or in those who find medication to be undesirable or intolerable, surgical management may be appropriate.

With appropriate patient selection, ambulatory surgery can be achieved for several surgical techniques. Patients identified as appropriate for day-case surgery must have good functional status confirmed at pre-operative assessment and an appropriate home situation upon discharge.

For procedures requiring a post-operative catheter (e.g., Rezūm, TURP, or holmium laser enucleation of prostate [HoLEP]), careful planning of catheter management is required. Patients require adequate training in catheter care and require access to medical support in case of difficulties and arrangements for removal.

Choice of anaesthetic plays an important role in the ability of a surgeon to offer a day case operation. With so many of our patients being elderly, the use of local or spinal anaesthesia reduces the risk of cognitive impairment, which can be problematic for this population after a general anaesthetic.

Transurethral Resection of Prostate (TURP)

Perhaps the most widely known prostate operation and historically the gold standard, a transurethral resection of prostate (TURP) involves the removal of benign adenoma in order to create a good urethral channel. A TURP may be performed either using a monopolar loop with glycine containing solution as the irrigant, or using a bipolar loop with saline as the irrigant (also known as transurethral resection on saline [TURIS]). A three-way catheter is placed post-operatively for irrigation and control of haematuria.

Traditionally, surgeons were concerned about the risk of TURP syndrome, a triad of hyponatremia, hypervolemia, and hyperammonaemia. This occurred as a consequence of the absorption of glycine resulting in diluted serum sodium levels, increased serum fluid levels, and the metabolism of glycine into ammonia causing encephalopathy. The advent of TURIS has almost eliminated this risk, and now, with careful post-operative irrigation and good out-of hospital access to post-operative advice, many centres successfully offer an ambulatory TURIS service.

Risks that should be highlighted to the patient are the risk of infection (1%), risk of blood transfusion (1%), incontinence (1%), retrograde ejaculation (60–70%), erectile dysfunction (10%). In selected patients it should be highlighted that if there is underlying detrusor failure, the procedure may not be 'successful' and, in general, for those with storage symptoms, one-third of patients will continue to experience some element of storage symptoms despite a 'successful' operation.

Urolift

For patients in whom sexual function is important, this minimally invasive procedure offers an improvement in voiding LUTS, with preservation of sexual function. Initially offered only to men with occlusive lateral lobes but no median lobe, an increasing number of studies have now shown good efficacy even in those with significant median lobes. Surgeons place implants to lift the enlarged prostatic tissue away from the urethra. Implants are placed in pairs, one on each lobe. The numbers of implants used directly correlated to the size and occlusive nature of the prostate.

There is persuasive 5- and 10-year data demonstrating sustained benefits, although it is widely acknowledged that many patients will require re-do surgery and that benefits seen are not as significant as with the more traditional surgeries such as TURP. Urolift is not always suitable for men with very large (>100 cc) prostates.

Rezūm

Rezūm uses radio-frequency energy to heat water, producing water vapour/steam. This water vapour is delivered into the tissue using a needle. Upon contact with the tissue the steam cools and condenses, and in doing so releases energy that damages the cell membranes, initiating cell necrosis.

The Rezūm convective water vapour treatment is also considered 'minimally invasive' and, although it is a newer technology, it is now starting to be performed under local anaesthesia.

Outcomes in terms of flow improvement and symptom improvement are comparable with trans-urethral resection, whilst impact on sexual function is highly unlikely; retrograde ejaculation risk is in the order of 2% and the risk of erectile dysfunction is less than 1%.

The procedure has the advantage of actually eliminating unwanted tissue and not requiring implantation of a foreign body. One downside is that the majority of patients require a two-way catheter for around four days post-operatively, but this is normally well tolerated with proper education.

Rezūm is already safely used in prostate volumes of up to 120 cc in some centres and is likely to become the treatment of choice for mild and moderate BPH in the future due to its ambulatory nature.

Laser Procedures: Holmium Laser Enucleation of Prostate (HoLEP)

Holmium Laser Enucleation of the Prostate is now considered the gold-standard surgical management for very large prostate glands (>120 cc). An anatomical enucleation of the tissues of the transitional zone is achieved with a combination of blunt dissection using the resectoscope and laser energy to encourage tissue separation and cauterise vessels. Risks are comparable with TURP, albeit with slightly lower rates of erectile dysfunction (likely owing to the lack of conducted electricity).

During HoLEP the enucleated prostatic adenoma is pushed into the bladder where it is morcellated using a nephroscope via the outer resectoscope sheath for vision. Morcellation should be performed carefully so as to not injure the bladder.

Photo vaporisation of the prostate (PVP), also known as potassium titanyl phosphate (KTP) laser vaporisation, uses a YAG laser shone through a potassium titanyl phosphate crystal to produce green light. This is preferentially taken up by haemoglobin and used to vaporise prostatic tissue. Surgeons performing high numbers of these procedures typically achieve excellent results, but the procedure has seen a decline in popularity amongst some surgeons in the last decade. PVP has been shown to be safe in patients taking anti-coagulation and anti-platelet medications, offering a clear superiority over some other techniques.

Both procedures can be performed under either general or spinal anaesthetic. Providing men are happy to be discharged with a catheter, this operation is amenable to a day case or a '23-hour' stay.

Other

The preceding list is by no means exhaustive. Open trans-vesical prostate enucleation is now largely regarded as a historic procedure, but newer technologies such as aquablation are garnering interest and could find a place in BPO surgical repertoire in the future. For the urologist looking to maximise the proportion of care delivered as ambulatory, the 'minimally invasive' techniques detailed earlier are the best means to achieve this.

Choice of Surgery

The choice of surgery will undoubtedly be dependent on the availability in your hospital. Patients should be encouraged to pursue day-case options where suitable. Factors influencing decision-making will include whether the patient is catheterised, indication for surgery (patients with refractory haematuria will require TURP or HoLEP), size of prostate, IPSS score, and patient choice.

Further Reading

Barry, M.J., Fowkler, F.J., O'Leary, M.P. et al. (1992). The American urological association symptom index for benign prostatic hyperplasia. *J. Urol.* 148: 1549–1557.

Cynk, M. (2014). Holmium laser enucleation of the prostate: a review of the clinical trial evidence. *Ther. Adv. Urol.* 6 (2): 62–73.

McVary, K.T. and Roehrborn, C.G. (2018). Three-year outcomes of the prospective randomized control Rezūm system study. *Urology* 111: 1–9.

Roehrborn, C.G., Siami, P., Barkin, J. et al. (2010). The effects of combination therapy with dutasteride and tamsulosin on clinical outcomes in men with symptomatic benign prostatic hyperplasia: 4-year results from the CombAT study. *Eur. Urol.* 51 (1): 123–131.

16

Urethral Catheters and Ambulatory Management of Urinary Retention

Ashiv Patel

The management of urinary retention is one of importance, particularly as most patients presenting with urinary retention can be managed using an 'ambulatory' model.

Urinary retention occurs most frequently in men over the age of 60, with this risk increasing with age. Males are 13 times more likely to be affected by acute urinary retention (AUR) than women. Over a five-year period, 10% of men over 70 will develop AUR whilst 30% of men over 80 will be affected.

An ambulatory approach will result in a reduced financial burden, better utilisation of inpatient beds and an improvement in patient-based outcomes through a reduction in admissions.

Risk Factors

Aside from advancing age, the presence of lower urinary tract symptoms (LUTS), larger prostate volume and previous spontaneous retention are all considered risk factors for urinary retention in men.

Definition of Acute Urinary Retention

Acute urinary retention (AUR) is defined as a painful inability to pass urine, followed by relief on draining the bladder through utilising a catheter. It is normally associated with >500 ml of urine being drained.

AUR can be classified as either being spontaneous or precipitated by an event. If the precipitating cause (e.g., infection) is treated, the retention usually resolves; however, spontaneous retention usually requires more definitive management.

Ambulatory Urology and Urogynaecology, First Edition. Edited by Abhay Rane and Ajay Rane.
© 2021 John Wiley & Sons Ltd. Published 2021 by John Wiley & Sons Ltd.

Definition of Chronic Urinary Retention

Defined as a non-painful bladder that is still palpable after voiding and post-void residual volumes in excess of 300 ml being present within the bladder.

Definition of Acute-on-Chronic Retention

Defined as a painful inability to pass urine, followed by relief on draining the bladder through utilising a catheter. It is normally associated with bladder volumes far in excess of 500 ml, typically 1000 ml or more.

Causes of Urinary Retention

Prostatic Enlargement

Both benign and malignant prostatic enlargement can cause urinary retention. These patients commonly present with lower urinary tract symptoms (LUTS); however, they may present more acutely with urinary retention.

Urethral Strictures

Due to a narrowing of the urethra, an outflow obstruction can occur secondary to a stricture that results in urinary retention.

Constipation

Faecal constipation can cause urinary retention by obstructing the urethra.

Infection

Infection or inflammation of the bladder, urethra, or prostate can cause obstruction of the urethra and lead to urinary retention.

Haematuria leading to Clot Retention

Urinary retention is precipitated by the obstruction of the urethra by clots formed secondary to haematuria. Any amount of macroscopic haematuria can result in clot retention; however, the subset of patients at greatest risk are those without sufficient bladder irrigation post-operatively.

Drugs

Drugs can be a precipitating cause of urinary retention. Drugs that commonly cause urinary retention include anaesthetics, anticholinergics, and sympathomimetic agents.

Pain

Abdominal pain and associated pelvic floor contraction can make it difficult for patients to pass urine, and adequate analgesic control is important in order to allow the patient to pass urine.

Post-operative Retention

There are a number of risk factors for urinary retention post-operatively. These include surgery involving the anorectum or perineum, bladder over-distension, instrumentation of the lower urinary tract, the use of epidural anaesthesia, and immobility in the post-operative period.

Pelvic Fracture and Urethral Injury

Pelvic fracture and urethral injury will cause urinary retention because the urine is unable to pass down a disrupted urethra.

Neurological Conditions (Parkinson's Disease, Multiple Sclerosis, Fowler's Syndrome)

Conditions that cause central nervous system disfunction can cause detrusor areflexia or detrusor sphincter dyssynergia. Fowler's syndrome is thought to cause impaired relaxation of the external urethral sphincter and can also cause urinary retention.

Cauda Equina

Cauda equina compression can be caused by a prolapsed lumbar disc, trauma, and benign or malignant masses. Compression or damage to the S2–S4 nerve roots can result in areflexia of the detrusor muscles and ultimately urinary retention.

Prolapse in Women

Women with cystoceles can suffer from urinary retention if the cystocele obstructs or creates a kink in the urethra. A vaginal support pessary provides a simple solution to correct anatomical position and relieve the issue.

Pelvic Masses

Pelvic masses can cause obstruction of the urethra and result in outflow obstruction and urinary retention.

Post-surgery for Stress Incontinence

Injury to the pelvic plexus can cause loss of motor innervation of the detrusor muscle and ultimately urinary retention.

Post-obstructive Diuresis

Defined as a condition of increased urine production of >200 ml for two consecutive hours following relief of retention or a total of 3000 ml over 24 hours.

Post-obstructive diuresis is a possibility when over 1000 ml is drained from the bladder using a catheter. This is a result of solute and fluid accumulation occurring due to prolonged renal obstruction, leading to a diuresis and polyuria through multiple mechanisms.

Post-obstructive diuresis will normally cease once homeostasis is achieved, but can become pathological and may cause electrolyte abnormalities, hypotension, dehydration leading to hypovolaemic shock and even death. Typical supportive management includes replacing 50% of the urine output by volume with intravenous fluids, but if the patient can freely drink according to their thirst, this can be a more physiologically accurate way of achieving the correct rate of fluid replacement in less severe diuresis.

Clinical Assessment of a Patient with Urinary Retention

Taking a full history and examination are central to the initial management of a patient with urinary retention. The most important factors to identify when taking a history from the patient include:

- Symptoms of prostatic enlargement: Frequency, urgency, nocturia, hesitancy, poor stream, intermittent flow, terminal dribbling.
- Symptoms of infection: Frequency, urgency, dysuria, visible haematuria.
- Constipation.
- Presence of visible clots and haematuria.
- Recent operative procedures, particularly those involving epidural and spinal anaesthesia.

- Symptoms of neurological conditions: Lower limb weakness, saddle anaesthesia, paraesthesia, faecal incontinence.
- Medications history: Anticholinergics, opiates, anti-histamines, tricyclic antidepressants.

Important factors when examining a patient with urinary retention are examination of the abdomen for a palpable bladder and performing a digital rectal exam in order to ascertain whether prostatic enlargement is a contributing factor in men.

It is paramount to make sure that the drained volume and fluid balance is clearly documented for any patient with urinary retention, particularly in those patients who drain more than 1000 ml of urine when a catheter is inserted. The patient's urine should also be tested using urine dip and sent for culture if positive.

Blood tests to monitor the patient's urea and electrolytes is also of key importance in order to correct any subsequent electrolyte abnormalities, before they become life threatening.

Catheter Insertion

Types of Urethral Catheters

Indwelling urethral catheters are composed of a semi-rigid tube that blocks the urethra but drains the bladder, they involve multiple lumens, with one controlled by an external valve that allows for the inflation of a balloon to maintain the catheters position in the bladder. Indwelling catheters can be broadly divided into two types; two-way catheters and three-way catheters. Two-way catheters are used for all types of urinary retention; three-way catheters are reserved for patients who require irrigation of their bladders either after suffering from clot retention secondary to haematuria or post-operatively.

Indwelling catheters come in a range of sizes and are described by the term 'French'. This relates to the catheters external circumference and was devised by the Parisian manufacturer of surgical instruments, Joseph-Frédéric-Benoît Charrière. Therefore, both two-way and three-way catheters will have the same external diameter if they have the same 'French' size. However, the three-way catheter will have the smaller drainage lumen, given the space occupied by the irrigation lumen.

Both two-way and three-way catheters have a further sub-type, which comes with a curved tip called either a Coudé tip or Tiemann tip catheter. This curved tip helps the catheter navigate any areas of constriction particularly constriction caused by an enlarged prostate in men.

Catheter Insertion Technique

Verbal consent is imperative to obtain from the patient, and this involves explaining the need for a catheter as well as what a catheter insertion will involve. The smallest sized catheter that will provide adequate drainage should be used.

The technique utilised is aseptic. Sterile water or saline should be used to prepare the skin around the urethral meatus. Lubricant jelly should then be applied to the urethra and this typically contains local anaesthetic. The catheter should be inserted until the flow of urine confirms it is situated in the bladder. The catheter balloon can then be inflated; however, care must be taken not to inflate the balloon whilst it is intra-urethral because this may cause damage to the patient's urethra and even urethral rupture.

The absence of urinary flow from the catheter indicates either the catheter is not in the bladder or that the diagnosis of urinary retention is incorrect.

In men, a curved-tip catheter can be used in order to facilitate entry of the catheter into the bladder. However, if the catheter will not pass into the bladder and it is certain that the patient is in urinary retention, then a flexible cystoscopy guided catheter insertion or supra-pubic catheter insertion is the next step in management. In extremis, a supra-pubic needle aspiration of urine can be used to drain enough urine to improve the patient's comfort whilst arrangements are put in place for a more definitive solution.

Flexible Cystoscopy Guided Catheter Insertion

If a flexible cystoscope is available, this should be the first choice when faced with a difficult catheterisation where a catheter cannot be placed into the bladder.

The flexible cystoscope can be used to enter the bladder under vision and site a guide-wire into the bladder. A catheter (an open Council-tip catheter for example) can then be 'rail-roaded' over the guide wire to achieve drainage.

Suprapubic Catheter Insertion

There are several things to consider before attempting supra-pubic catheterisation. Whether the patient may have bladder cancer and the risk of spread through the created tract, previous abdominal surgery that may have caused adhesions, pelvic fractures, and the presence of a pelvic haematoma, anticoagulation, vascular graft in situ in the pelvic region.

Antibiotic prophylaxis is recommended if there is a concurrent urine infection. Abdominal examination to check for a distended bladder and a BAUS (British Association of Urological Surgeons) recommended ultrasound to identify any interposing bowel in the planned tract. Commence with aspiration of urine using a 21G needle, 2 cm superior to the pubic symphysis.

The suprapubic trocar should then be placed 2 cm above the pubic symphysis and inserted following infiltration of local anaesthetic in the same direction that urine was aspirated.

Patients with Urinary Retention requiring Admission

Patients with chronic or acute-on-chronic urinary retention must be considered for admission to monitor their urine output for post obstructive diuresis and blood tests the following day to assess for any electrolyte abnormalities.

Any patient with a difficult catheterisation requiring the use of flexible cystoscopy guidance or the insertion of a suprapubic catheter should be admitted to hospital for monitoring and a decision on definitive treatment.

Ambulatory Urology and Urinary Retention

Patients with a simple ambulatory urinary retention (AUR) (500–800 ml drained volume) will usually be manageable in an ambulatory fashion. Once the precipitating cause is identified and reversed following the insertion of a catheter, the patient can be safely discharged if there are no abnormalities on blood tests and they are not in diuresis. They can be seen in urology outpatients or in a trial-without-catheter clinic in order to further assess their needs and the next steps in their management.

The 'outpatient' catheter service requires careful planning in order to be able to prevent the need for the patient to re-attend prior to the planned catheter removal and avoid unnecessary stress and anxiety for the patient. This involves adequate explanation and education of catheter care prior to discharge and the means for the patient to have a point-of-contact within the department in case of difficulties or need for supplies. Catheter removal should be timed for a point that minimises indwelling catheter time (thus reducing risk of infection) whilst allowing sufficient time for recovery to optimise chances of successful voiding. For the majority of male AUR, two weeks is considered the standard catheter indwelling time. Medication such as tamsulosin (further discussed in the prostatic obstruction chapter) can lower bladder outlet resistance and maximise chances of success.

Further Reading

Fisher, E., Subramonian, K., Omar, M.I. et al. (2014). The role of alpha blockers prior to removal of urethral catheter for acute urinary retention in men. *Cochrane Database Syst. Rev.* 6: Cd006744.

Gonzalez, C.M. (2004). Pathophysiology, diagnosis, and treatment of the post obstructive diuresis. In: *Management of Benign Prostatic Hypertrophy* (ed. M.V. KT), 35–45. New York: Humana Press.

Gravas S., Cornu JN., Gacci M. et al. (2019). EAU Guidelines on the management of non-neurogenic male lower urinary tract symptoms. European Association of Urology. http://uroweb.org/guideline/treatment-of-non-neurogenic-male-luts.

Harrison, S.C.W., Lawrence, W.T., Morley, R. et al. (2010). British Association of Urological Surgeons' suprapubic catheter practice guidelines. *BJU Int.* 107 (1): 77–85.

17

Paediatric Urology

Tharani Nitkunan and Sylvia Yan

Much like adult urology, a focused history and examination should be taken from the child and parents/caregiver to aid diagnosis and management in paediatric urology. In this section, we will aim to discuss clinical investigations and management of paediatric urological conditions commonly seen in the clinic setting.

Recurrent Urinary Tract Infections

Urinary tract infections (UTIs) are the most common bacterial infection in the paediatric population. The incidence is initially higher in boys, affecting up to 20.3% of uncircumcised boys and 5% of girls at the age of 1. There is a gradual shift, with UTIs affecting 3% of prepubertal girls and 1% of prepubertal boys. The National Institute for Health and Care Excellence (NICE) have defined a recurrent UTI as two or more episodes of pyelonephritis, or one episode of pyelonephritis plus one or more episodes of cystitis, or three or more episodes of cystitis.

Diagnostic investigations include urinalysis, which may require suprapubic bladder aspiration or bladder catheterisation in infants. A urine culture and microscopy should be carried out if there is evidence of infection. The role of further imaging is to differentiate between an uncomplicated and complicated UTI, but should also be considered in those with haematuria. A UTI is complicated in the presence of an abnormal urinary tract including upper tract dilatation, atrophic or duplex kidneys, ureterocoele, posterior urethral valves, intestinal connections, and vesico-ureteric reflux (VUR). NICE guidelines recommend an urgent ultrasound of the urinary tract for all those with recurrent UTI under six months. For children six months and older, NICE in the UK recommends an

Ambulatory Urology and Urogynaecology, First Edition. Edited by Abhay Rane and Ajay Rane.
© 2021 John Wiley & Sons Ltd. Published 2021 by John Wiley & Sons Ltd.

ultrasound within six weeks of the latest infective episode. All children with recurrent UTIs should be referred to a paediatric specialist and have a dimercapto-succinic acid (DMSA) scan within four to six months of an acute infection to evaluate for renal scarring. European Association of Urology (EAU) guidelines recommend a renal tract ultrasound in febrile UTIs if there is no clinical improvement, as an abnormal result is seen in 15% of these patients.

Antimicrobial treatment for each episode should be guided by the local antimicrobial guidelines to avoid contributing to resistance. In principle, antibiotic prophylaxis should not be prescribed following a first episode of UTI. In those with recurrent UTIs, trimethoprim and nitrofurantoin are the recommended first line antibiotics by NICE. If unsuitable or second line treatment is needed, cephalexin and amoxicillin should be considered. This should be reviewed on a regular basis and behavioural, personal hygiene measures and self-care treatments should always be discussed prior to antibiotic prophylaxis.

Reflux

Vesico-ureteric reflux is a common cause of complicated UTIs and is seen in up to 50% of children presenting with UTIs. The incidence is higher in boys (29%) compared to girls (14%) and they also tend to have higher grades of VUR. Although it can be asymptomatic, VUR is seen in 16.2% of those found to have hydronephrosis in-utero. There is a hereditary risk, in those with parents with VUR having an incidence of 35.7%, and a 22% sibling risk.

Basic investigations should include a detailed history to establish risk factors, clinical examination with blood pressure assessment, urinalysis to evaluate for proteinuria, urine culture, and serum creatinine, if indicated. Imaging such as an ultrasound of kidneys and bladder will evaluate for evidence of hydronephrosis. Diagnosis of VUR is made on voiding cystourethrography (VCUG), which also allows assessment of the grade of reflux (Table 17.1) and bladder and urethral configuration. A DMSA nuclear medicine scan can be considered at baseline to detect any renal scarring and as a comparison for subsequent future imaging. In concurrence, lower urinary tract assessment is essential; it is known that treating lower urinary tract dysfunction (LUTD) can aid resolution of VUR.

For infants presenting with hydronephrosis diagnosed on antenatal scanning, ultrasound of the urinary tract is the recommended imaging modality to commence with. This is usually done after the first week of birth, as there is a period of oliguria in the neonate. Two normal successive post-natal ultrasound examinations within two months of life is reassuring, indicating that if there is any VUR, it is likely to be of low grade. If ultrasound reveals any cortical abnormality or signs of LUTD, then a VCUG would be recommended for further evaluation.

Table 17.1 Grading system for VUR on VCUG, according to the International Reflux Study Committee.

Grade I	Reflux does not reach the renal pelvis; varying degrees of ureteric dilatation
Grade II	Reflux reaches the renal pelvis; no dilatation of the collecting system; normal fornices
Grade III	Mild to moderate dilatation of the ureter, with or without kinking; moderated dilatation of the collecting system; normal or minimally deformed fornices
Grade IV	Moderate dilatation of the ureter with or without kinking; moderate dilatation of the collecting system; blunt fornices, but impressions of the papillae still visible
Grade V	Gross dilatation and kinking of the ureter, marked dilatation of the collecting system; papillary impressions not visible, intraparenchymal reflux

Source: Adapted from Tekgül et al. (2012).

Table 17.2 Percentage of patients found to have spontaneous resolution of VUR in accordance to grade of VUR.

	% spontaneous resolution with 4–5 years of follow-up
Grade I – II	80%
Grade III – V	30–50%

Source: Modified from Tekgül et al. (2012).

Treatment for VUR is dependent on the grade of reflux and symptoms such as febrile UTIs. Parameters that are favourable for spontaneous resolution include age of less than one year at time of presentation, male gender, grade I–III reflux, and asymptomatic presentation. In those with unilateral grade I–II reflux, patient and parents can be reassured there is up to 80% likelihood that there will be complete resolution of VUR by five years (Table 17.2). As previously suggested, treatment for LUTD, such as a circumcision in those with VUR and UTI is recommended because it may lead to resolution of VUR.

Regular follow up with imaging and symptom review is the mainstay of conservative treatment. There is no current guideline on frequency of imaging, but EAU guidelines recommend biannual ultrasound scans of the renal tract with annual cystography and DMSA scans. In patients with a history of UTI or recurrent UTI and high grade of reflux, antibiotic prophylaxis should be administered. Amoxicillin and trimethoprim are recommended for those less than two months and trimethoprim-sulfamethoxazole or nitrofurantoin can be used in older infants.

Although there is no clear evidence regarding the suitable duration of prophylaxis, some trials suggest a renal protective effect in those with VUR having prophylaxis.

Failing conservative treatment, surgical options include endoscopic sub ureteral bulking injections and ureteric reimplantation. Bulking agents can be injected submucosally inferior to the intramural portion of the ureter to increase coaptation. This success rates are in the range of 78.5%, 72%, 63,% and 52% for grades I, II, III, and IV reflux, respectively. Various techniques have been described for paediatric ureteric reimplantation, with laparoscopic approaches being adopted in some centres. They have all been reported to have excellent success rates between 92 and 98%.

Undescended Testes

Cryptorchidism, or undescended testes (UDT), affects up to 4.6% of full-term male infants and they remain undescended in 1% of boys by age 1. The classification for UDT is mainly categorised into palpable and non-palpable testes (Table 17.3). History and clinical examination (supine and standing positions) is crucial for assessing for UDT. Careful examination with sweeping warm fingers along the inguinal canal towards the pubic tubercle can occasionally allow palpation of the inguinal UDT. It is also important to examine the common areas for ectopic testes including the superficial inguinal pouch, femoral, perineal, pubic, penile, or contralateral side. There is currently no role for imaging in the diagnostic evaluation

Table 17.3 Classification of undescended testes.

Undescended testes	Palpable	Inguinal
		Ectopic
		• Superficial inguinal pouch
		• Femoral
		• Perineal
		• Pubic
		• Penile
		• Contralateral
		Retractile
	Non-palpable	Inguinal
		Ectopic
		Intra-abdominal
		Absent
	Acquired/re-ascended	

Source: Adapted from Radmayr et al. (2016).

of UDT. Retractile testes carry a 7–32% risk of re-ascent and should be followed up clinically on an annual basis until puberty.

It is rare for the UDT to descend after 6 months of age; therefore, the current British Association for Paediatric Urologists recommends treatment to be complete by 12 months as transformation of germ cells are usually complete by this time point. The EAU guidelines extend this up to 18 months at the latest. For palpable UDT, an examination under anaesthetic (EUA) and inguinal orchidopexy is the widely accepted surgical approach with a 92% success rate. Parents should be warned of the risks of postoperative testicular atrophy and risk of re-ascent.

For those with non-palpable testes, a EUA is the first step of treatment. If under anaesthetic, the testis is identified, an inguinal orchidopexy could be undertaken. If the testis is still not identified, proceeding to inguinal exploration or a diagnostic laparoscopy with either subsequent orchidectomy or orchidolysis and orchidopexy as is appropriate. Seventy-five percent of testes identified laparoscopically will be viable, with some cases requiring a two-stage Fowler-Stephens approach, which carries an 80% success rate. Orchidopexy for the contralateral testis is recommended. These cases are usually conducted by a specialist paediatric urologist at a dedicated paediatric unit.

Some patients may present post-pubertally with an UDT. A previous study with 51 men presenting with a unilateral inguinal UDT and a normal contralateral testis demonstrated that the incidence of intratubular germ cell neoplasia in the UDT was 2%. In this group of patients, they should be counselled regarding risk of malignancy and benefits of orchidopexy or orchidectomy.

Patients and parents will often enquire about the impact of UDT on fertility and risk of malignancy. It is known that early surgical intervention will reduce the impact on germ cell and Leydig cell loss. Following surgical treatment of unilateral UDT, the fertility rate remains lower than those with bilateral descended testes. However, the paternity rate remains comparable. For those with treated bilateral UDT, both the fertility and paternity rates are lower. The principle for early surgical intervention applies to the risk of testicular malignancy. A study of 17 000 patients found that the relative risk of testicular cancer in those treated before age 13 was twofold, compared to those treated after age 13 with a risk more than fivefold. Patients and parents should be fully counselled about the above risks, and patients should be encouraged to undertake regular self-examination.

Phimosis

In the paediatric clinic, this is a very common presentation and much of it is in the counselling of the natural history of the foreskin. During the first year of age, only 50% of boys will have a retractile foreskin. This increases to 92% by age 7 and by age 16, only 1% of boys will be troubled by phimosis.

Current indications for circumcision are pathological phimosis with evidence of lichen sclerosis of the foreskin, 3 or more episodes of recurrent balanoposthitis within 6–12 months and recurrent febrile UTIs, and an abnormal urinary tract (complicated UTIs). Establishing the occurrence of balanoposthitis can be challenging and a focused history is key. Balanoposthitis is inflammation of the glans and prepuce, which is speculated to be secondary to irritation from the breakdown of urea in urine, liberating ammonia.

For those that do not require a circumcision, foreskin care advice and reassurance regarding the natural history of the foreskin is advised. To prevent episodes of balanoposthitis, parents should be advised to continue with simple bathing with avoidance of perfumed soaps. The foreskin can be gently retracted on a regular basis and dabbing post-voiding will help reduce the risk of urinary trapping and irritation. During a flare of balanoposthitis, topical steroids and antibiotics should be used. Discussing the criteria for circumcision can aid in follow-up planning and allows parents to look out for any change in condition that may require re-referral for surgical intervention.

Enuresis

This is a common condition, affecting up to 10% of children attending school. There is a reported association with constipation, obstructive airway disease, obesity, and behavioural disorders such as attention deficit disorder and autism spectrum disorder. Enuresis can be divided into primary (those who have never been dry) and secondary enuresis (those that have previously had a period of six months or more of being dry). In secondary enuresis, it is important to identify any potential psychological or social trigger. Enuresis is also further classified into monosymptomatic (MEN) and non-monosymptomatic (NMEN) enuresis. Patients with NMEN will present with associated urinary symptoms such as UTIs, stress urinary incontinence (SUI) or even signs of ectopic ureters.

Important things to elicit in the history and examination include daytime voiding symptoms, suggestions of Vincent's curtsey (indicator of overactive bladder), whether the patient is a deep sleeper, examination of bladder, external genitalia, and signs of spinal abnormalities. First line investigations include urinalysis to exclude infection and a bladder and bowel diary. A child's bladder capacity in millilitres can be calculated by the formula $= (age \times 30) + 30$. Ultrasound scan be used for patients with suspected congenital malformations and those refractory to initial treatment. It can also obtain a post void residual urine volume.

Treatment is recommended in a step-wise approach, starting with fluid and stool charts if applicable. The child and parents should be encouraged to ensure adequate hydration and good urinary habits, especially at school. For MEN, alarm systems can be used, providing up to 80% success rate. The use of desmopressin can be considered and if there is a particular event that the child/parent would like the child to be dry for, it is recommended to commence treatment in the two weeks leading up to it. The success rate is quoted at 70% but has a high relapse rate, unlike the alarm system. Dosage starts at 120 mcg and can be increased to 240 mcg. There is no risk of hyponatraemia.

Patients with NMEN should have their daytime symptoms addressed, and if there is evidence of overactive bladder, antimuscarinics such as oxybutynin, tolterodine, and solifenacin can be used.

Enuresis can be stressful for the child and their families, and if there is no response to treatment, any missed comorbidities, anatomical, or functional causes should be examined for.

Further Reading

Gairdner, D. (1949). The fate of the foreskin, a study of circumcision. *Br. Med. J.* 2: 1433–1437.

Haid, B. and Tekgül, S. (2017). Primary and secondary enuresis: pathophysiology, diagnosis, and treatment. *Eur. Urol. Focus* 3: 198–206.

Okarska-Napierała, M., Wasilewska, A., Kuchar, E. et al. (2017). Urinary tract infection in children: diagnosis, treatment, imaging – comparison of current guidelines. *J. Pediatr. Urol.* 13 (6): 567–573.

Radmayr, C., Dogan, H., Hoebeke, P. et al. (2016). EAU guideline for management of undescended testes: European Association of Urology/European Society for Paediatric Urology Guidelines. *J. Pediatr. Urol.* 12 (6): 335–343.

Tekgül, S., Riedmiller, H., Hoebeke, P. et al. (2012). EAU guidelines on vesicoureteral reflux in children. *Eur. Urol.* 62 (3): 534–542.

18

Urothelial Bladder Cancer

Diagnosis and Management in the Outpatient Clinic

Jordan Durrant

Bladder Cancer Investigation

Due to the concerning nature of haematuria for patients and the value of making an early diagnosis, the concept of 'One-Stop' clinics for the investigation of suspected urothelial bladder cancer is now well established.

A 'One-Stop' service will normally aim to offer a patient all the necessary investigations with the minimum number of hospital attendances possible, with everything ideally being done for the patient on the same day. On receipt of a referral of a patient with haematuria, a urology department will normally organise:

- Upper Urinary Tract Imaging
- Clinical Assessment – urine dipstick test, history, and examination
- Flexible Cystoscopy
- Urine Cytology in some circumstances

Upper urinary tract imaging is normally dependent on the nature of the haematuria. Non-visible haematuria (NVH) (microscopic haematuria) is investigated with a renal tract ultrasound scan, whereas visible (macroscopic) haematuria is investigated with a computerized tomography intravenous urogram (CT IVU), including excretory phase urography). This is based on the fact that visible haematuria (as compared to non-visible) confers virtually twice the risk of finding an underlying urothelial tumour.

Clinical Assessment

Initial assessment requires determination of the type of haematuria:

- Visible haematuria
- Persistent non-visible haematuria on multiple tests
- Symptomatic non-visible haematuria (associated with pain or lower urinary tract symptoms)

Ambulatory Urology and Urogynaecology, First Edition. Edited by Abhay Rane and Ajay Rane.
© 2021 John Wiley & Sons Ltd. Published 2021 by John Wiley & Sons Ltd.

Careful history-taking is valuable, particularly in cases of symptomatic NVH, in order to determine whether urinary tract infections are a potential cause of the haematuria. Urine dipstick testing will help to identify patients with ongoing signs of infection; however, review of previous MSU microscopy and culture results, if available, can be more useful.

Urine dipstick testing also allows detection of proteinuria. This finding then requires further clarification with protein-creatinine ratio testing but an abnormal level (>50 mg/mmol) can indicate the cause of haematuria being glomerulonephritis, IgA nephropathy, or another nephrological condition requiring renal medicine/nephrology specialist input.

Initial physical examination may suggest an underlying pathology – a ballotable renal mass may suggest renal cell cancer, a distended bladder may suggest bladder outflow obstruction and associated urinary tract infection (UTI). An abnormal prostate on digital rectal examination (DRE) is indicative of prostate cancer.

Particular attention should be paid to any history of tobacco usage and smoking as this may influence levels of suspicion and prompt more rigorous investigation (CT scanning or urine cytology) on the basis of the increased risk of urothelial cancer.

Cystoscopy

Ideally, the patient will attend for flexible cystoscopy after completion of necessary upper tract imaging. If imaging clearly demonstrates a urothelial bladder cancer, flexible cystoscopy is rarely required and the patient should instead be counselled to proceed directly to trans-urethral resection in the operating theatre at the earliest opportunity.

Flexible cystoscopy is carried out using flexible fibre-optic flexible cystoscopes with the use of intra-urethral lidocaine lubricant. Use of a full syringe of anaesthetic lubricant in females is not necessary and risks obscuring vision in the bladder. In male patients, it has been demonstrated that cooled anaesthetic lubricant is associated with less discomfort on instillation, as is very slow instillation of the lubricant also. Studies have indicated that maximum analgesic effect from lidocaine lubricant occurs after an indwelling time of >15 minutes, this is impractical in most haematuria clinics however.

Most urology departments have an adopted policy of deferring flexible cystoscopy in the event of signs of a urine infection being found on urine dipstick testing. Midstream urine specimen (MSU) is sent for microscopy, culture, and sensitivity and empirical antibiotics are commenced, and the cystoscopy is rebooked for a later date. It is important to be aware that almost 50% of bladder tumours are colonised by bacteria, and persistent infection despite antibiotic treatment must not be allowed to lead to repeated deferral and delayed diagnosis in such cases. If such a scenario is a concern, then proceeding with flexible cystoscopy whilst giving antibiotic cover (e.g. IV gentamicin) may be the best course of action, if safe to do so.

Further Steps

Ideally a 'complete' set of investigations for haematuria should include blood tests (including renal function testing) and urine cytology. Availability of urine cytology is variable, however, and in some cases it's use may be restricted to patients with visible haematuria only. Urine cytology is only a reliable indicator of high-grade disease.

Patients with a confirmed finding of a bladder tumour in clinic should be offered trans-urethral resection for definitive diagnosis, and a staging CT scan should ideally be arranged prior to this. For patients with NVH but a positive smoking history that prompts a high level of clinical suspicion, it may be prudent to organise CT urography for further reassurance.

Further support to the patient should ideally be made available at this stage from a member of the cancer team (e.g. a cancer nurse specialist).

Transurethral Resection of a Bladder Tumour Surgery

In most cases, transurethral resection of a bladder tumour (TURBT) surgery will require an overnight stay with an indwelling catheter for the patient, but smaller tumours may allow same-day discharge of the patient. In cases of apparent superficial tumour, intravesical Mitomycin C as a single post-operative dose has been shown to result in a relative risk reduction of recurrence by 39%. If systems and protocols are in place for this to be administered in the operating theatre at the end of the procedure or in the anaesthetic recovery area, this can still allow drainage of Mitomycin and removal of the catheter one hour later to facilitate same-day discharge.

Risk Stratification and Further Treatment and Follow-Up for Non-muscle Invasive Disease

Histological analysis of a TURBT specimen, in conjunction with radiological staging, allows determination of whether the urothelial bladder cancer is muscle invasive, or non-muscle invasive. This is the most significant factor determining future care. Failure to sample detrusor muscle at the time of surgery should immediately prompt a repeat TURBT procedure after six weeks. Histology and scan results should be discussed at a multi-disciplinary team meeting so that treatment planning can take place.

Low Risk

Patients with pTa G1 (<3 cm), pTa G2 low (<3 cm) and papillary urothelial neoplasm of low malignant potential (PUNLMP) are stratified because low-risk will be recommended to have a flexible cystoscopy at 3 months and 12 months following initial diagnosis. Evidence suggests that these patients can be safely discharged at the end of one year, and this is current UK practice. Urine cytology is not useful in the follow-up of low-risk disease.

Intermediate Risk

Patients with intermediate risk will be offered a six-dose course of intravesical Mitomycin C. It should be explained that a course of Mitomycin C is associated with a relative risk reduction in recurrence rate of 11%. Side effects include urinary tract infection, bladder irritation/pain, and dysuria. Neutropenia is a very rare side effect.

Recurrence following six weeks' intravesical Mitomycin C is concerning and should prompt re-discussion in a multidisciplinary team (MDT) setting. Cystoscopic surveillance is usually offered on a reducing schedule and UK guidelines recommend cystoscopy at 3, 9, and 18 months from the time of diagnosis. Annual cystoscopy is offered thereafter.

Patients who have been followed up for at least five years can be considered discharge in selected cases. (e.g. Solitary G1 and G2 [low] disease with no recurrence and no ongoing tobacco use); however, individual urology units may have different approaches to this.

High Risk

Patients with a new diagnosis of high-risk non-muscle invasive disease should be offered a repeat TURBT (re-resection) at six weeks. These are patients with pTa G3, pT1 disease and carcinoma in situ (CIS). The rationale for re-resection is that it has been found that 75% of patients with high-risk disease have residual tumour at re-resection and 20% of those will have muscle-invasive disease. Furthermore, it is known that for disease that is not 'up-staged' on re-resection, the future risk of recurrence is halved after a six-week re-resection.

After cases of high-risk disease have been discussed at an MDT, patients will typically be offered a choice between intra-vesical immunotherapy using BCG (Bacillus Calmette-Guerin) or Radical Cystectomy surgery. Fifteen-year data shows that half of patients choosing BCG will experience progression, but just under one-third will survive with an intact bladder. Cystoscopic surveillance typically takes place at three-month intervals for the first two years, then six-month intervals for two years, and annual thereafter. Urine cytology can also be a useful tool for surveillance of high-grade disease.

Low Risk	Intermediate Risk	High Risk
pTa G1 <3 cm	pTa G1 >3 cm	pTa G3
pTa G2(low) <3 cm	pTa G1 **multifocal**	pT1 G2
PUNLMP	pTa G2(low) >3 cm	pT1 G3
	pTa G2(low) **multifocal**	pTis/CIS
	pTa G2(**high**)	micropapillary/nested
	pTa G2(grade not further stated)	
	Low-Risk **recurrence** within 12 months	

Muscle Invasive Disease

Patients with muscle invasive disease will be offered either radical radiotherapy or radical cystectomy surgery via an MDT. A number of protocols exist for radiotherapy, but mostly consist of fractions being delivered over the course of four to six weeks. The standard of care for radical cystectomy is to offer ileal conduit urinary diversion at the same time. Some centres offer continent urinary diversion in select cases, but this can be associated with higher complication rates and is generally reserved for highly motivated patients with minimal co-morbidities. With either treatment, outcomes over a five-year period are extremely similar with overall survival being 50–60%.

Further Reading

National Institute for Health and Care Excellence (2015). Bladder cancer: diagnosis and management. NICE guideline. (February 25, 2015). www.nice.org.uk/guidance/ng2.

19

Prostate Cancer

Diagnosis and Management in the Outpatient Clinic

David Thurtle

Prostate cancer is the commonest male solid organ malignancy. Approximately 50 000 men are diagnosed every year in the UK. Its prevalence and the high profile of the disease, means it represents a fair proportion of the workload for most practising adult urologists.

Most patients will first be referred with a raised prostate specific antigen (PSA) test. This simple and cheap blood test can lead to a multitude of investigations and treatments with significant potential morbidity, so it is important to be able to counsel men thoroughly. Unlike many cancers, some forms of non-metastatic prostate cancer can very reasonably be monitored by 'active surveillance' (AS) rather than requiring universal treatment – creating decision dilemmas for patients and clinicians and emphasising the importance of understanding the disease thoroughly.

Pathology

The vast majority of prostate cancer is adenocarcinoma – from the glandular structures in the epithelial tissue. Very rarely, the prostate can be a site for sarcomas or secondary metastases. Most prostate adenocarcinomas occur in the peripheral zone (~75%), whereas the transitional zone is more commonly affected by benign enlargement. Prostate cancer is usually considered to be a multifocal disease.

Two histological lesions have traditionally been considered to be pre- or peri-malignant lesions, namely, prostatic intraepithelial neoplasia (PIN) and atypical small acinar proliferation (ASAP). Only high-grade PIN (HGPIN) should be recorded by pathologists. Isolated HGPIN or ASAP may lead to repeated biopsies, or longer PSA monitoring, but does not in itself require treatment.

Tumour Grading

Prostate cancer is graded using the Gleason score (GS), composed of two scores ranging from 1 to 5 based upon the morphology of the dominant and the non-dominant cell pattern. Gleason score of 3 + 3 and above are considered to be cancer. In 2014 the International Society of Urological Pathologists published a revised cancer 'Grade Group' system which seeks to make the grading more intuitive – with grade groups 1 (GS 3 + 3), 2 (GS 3 + 4), 3 (GS 4 + 3), 4 (GS 8), and 5 (GS 9–10) ranging from the lowest to highest-risk disease.

Biopsy characteristics have prognostic significance, as a surrogate for disease volume and multifocality. Proportion of biopsy cores involved, maximum tumour length, and total biopsy percentage are sometimes used.

History

History-taking for a man suspected to have prostate cancer can be considered in two parts – risk factors for the disease and symptoms of the disease:

Risk Factors

Age – Prostate cancer prevalence increases with age. Incidence rates are highest in men aged between 75 and 79. The disease is very rare under the age of 40, whereas cadaveric studies have shown the prevalence to be in excess of 50% by age 80 – though much of this will not be indolent.

Hormones – Benign or malignant growth of the prostate is under the influence of testosterone and it's active metabolite dihydrotestosterone (DHT). Therefore, men who take additional testosterone may be at higher risk of the disease. Men on testosterone replacement therapy, tend to have their PSA monitored for this reason. Conversely, 5-alpha reductase inhibitors (5-ARI) (e.g., finasteride) have the effect of shrinking the prostate reducing PSA values. PSA values among men on 5-ARIs are usually doubled to compensate for this effect. Impact of long term 5-ARIs on prostate cancer is debated.

Race – The disease is more common and aggressive among black men than Caucasians. Men of Asian or Oriental origin tend to be at lower risk.

Family history – Carriers of the breast cancer susceptibility protein (BRCA) gene mutations are at increased risk, and may have more aggressive, prostate cancer. Family history should therefore enquire about breast and ovarian malignancies among relatives, as well as prostate cancer. Men with one first degree relative affected by prostate cancer are approximately twice as likely to develop prostate cancer, with the risk increasing with more affected relatives.

Obesity – Emerging research suggests obese men are at higher risk of prostate cancer, and have worse outcomes from the disease, with the effect thought to be multifactorial.

Diet and lifestyle – Prostate cancer is not thought to have a direct association with smoking. Some foods, such as lycopenes (e.g., tomatoes) and cruciferous vegetables (e.g., broccoli) are thought to have protective effects against prostate cancer.

Symptoms of the Disease

As prostate cancer tends to affect the peripheral zone of the prostate, it is often completely asymptomatic.

Lower urinary tract symptoms (LUTS) such as nocturia, frequency, hesitancy, urgency, or retention are more likely to be a result of benign prostatic enlargement, but can suggest underlying malignancy. Regardless, existing LUTS may have an impact on eventual treatment decisions. Primary care guidelines often suggest considering a PSA test in men with LUTS, as well as those with erectile dysfunction.

Haematuria and haematospermia, have been associated with prostate cancer, although more common causes for both exist. Isolated haematospermia is generally benign and self-limiting.

Symptoms of advanced disease may be more systemic, such as weight loss and lethargy. Localised extension can lead to perineal pain, renal failure and anuria and rarely even malignant priapism or rectal obstruction. Symptoms of bone metastases such as back pain, bone pain, anaemia, and neurological symptoms in the lower limbs suggest advanced disease.

Sex and fertility are important considerations, and erectile function should be documented, as potential treatments may affect these.

Examination and Investigation

In addition to a history, examination, and PSA, most new patients with PSA < ~30 are best investigated with upfront pre-biopsy multi-parametric magnetic resonance imaging (mpMRI) (see below). If subsequent biopsy demonstrates low-risk disease, further staging investigations can be omitted. For high-risk cases, bone scan and computed tomography (CT) are used for staging. A patient presenting with symptoms or high PSA (>50) suggestive of advanced disease could proceed directly to bone scan without need for an mpMRI.

Digital rectal examination (DRE) of the prostate is a quick and simple test that should not be omitted, although it is widely appreciated that correlation between DRE and MRI or pathological findings is poor. DRE can be useful to detect obviously malignant prostates, which tend to feel hard, fixed, craggy, nodular, and asymmetric. DRE can also help roughly quantify prostate volume to contextualise the PSA value, and to identify competing diagnoses such as a tender boggy prostate suggesting prostatitis.

PSA remains the mainstay for prostate cancer detection. It is specific to the prostate, but not to prostate cancer. PSA rises with increasing age and prostate size, hence the increasing interest in PSA-density (PSA/prostate volume). PSA is also raised by prostatitis or urinary tract infection, catheterisation, retention or instrumentation to the urinary tract. Patients are advised to avoid intercourse or cycling for a few days before a PSA test, which may also raise the PSA value to a lesser extent. In cases of infection or retention it is advisable to retest the PSA approximately six weeks later.

The PSA test measures the total of both free and bound PSA. There has been significant research interest in PSA-isoforms such as free-PSA and pro-PSA, or the ratios of free: total. The hope is that these may be more specific to prostate cancer itself, but none have yet become widely used in clinical practice. In undiagnosed men and those on surveillance, 'PSA kinetics' are of interest including PSA doubling time and PSA velocity.

Multiparametric MRI

Magnetic resonance imaging has been the biggest advance in prostate cancer management in recent years. 'Multiparametric' refers to the addition of at least one 'functional' sequence to the standard anatomical T1- and T2-weighted imaging. The most commonly used functional sequences are dynamic contrast enhanced (DCE) and diffusion-weighted imaging (DWI). Magnetic resonance spectroscopy is another example but is now rarely used. Magnetic resonance imaging should generally be reserved for those who might potentially be eligible for radical treatment.

Multiparametric magnetic resonance imaging (mpMRI) has two key roles in modern practice, first in detection and targeting, and second in staging (Table 19.1). Radiologists report MRI lesions on a five-point scale – most commonly version 2 of the PI-RADS (prostate imaging –reporting and data system) classification. Scores of 1, 3, and 5 suggest 'very low,' 'intermediate,' and 'very high' likelihood of clinically significant prostate cancer. Biopsy is generally offered to those with PIRADs score 3 or more, and can be omitted in those with a score of 1 or 2, after reaching a shared decision with the patient. MRI-staging can also be useful to inform surgical decision making – including whether to attempt a nerve-sparing

Table 19.1 Prostate cancer staging.

Clinical/Pathological Tumour Staging	Cancer Stage Grouping
TX: The primary tumour cannot be evaluated.	
T0 (T plus zero): There is no evidence of a tumour in the prostate	
T1: The tumour cannot be felt during a DRE and is not seen during imaging tests. It may be found when surgery is done for another reason, usually for BPH or an abnormal growth of noncancerous prostate cells. • **T1a:** The tumour is in 5% or less of the prostate tissue removed during surgery. • **T1b:** The tumour is in more than 5% of the prostate tissue removed during surgery. • **T1c:** The tumour is found during a needle biopsy, usually because the patient has an elevated PSA level.	**Stage I:** Cancer in this early stage is usually slow growing. The tumour cannot be felt and involves one-half of one side of the prostate or even less than that. PSA levels are low. The cancer cells are well differentiated, meaning they look like healthy cells (cT1a–cT1c or cT2a or pT2, N0, M0, PSA level is less than 10, Grade Group 1).
T2: The tumour is found only in the prostate, not other parts of the body. It is large enough to be felt during a DRE. • **T2a:** The tumour involves one-half of 1 side of the prostate. • **T2b:** The tumour involves more than one-half of 1 side of the prostate but not both sides. • **T2c:** The tumour has grown into both sides of the prostate.	**Stage II:** The tumour is found only in the prostate. PSA levels are medium or low. Stage II prostate cancer is small but may have an increasing risk of growing and spreading. • **Stage IIA:** The tumour cannot be felt and involves half of 1 side of the prostate or even less than that. PSA levels are medium, and the cancer cells are well differentiated (cT1a–cT1c or cT2a, N0, M0, PSA level is between 10 and 20, Grade Group 1). This stage also includes larger tumours confined to the prostate as long as the cancer cells are still well differentiated (cT2b–cT2c, N0, M0, PSA level is less than 20, Group 1). • **Stage IIB:** The tumour is found only inside the prostate, and it may be large enough to be felt during DRE. The PSA level is medium. The cancer cells are moderately differentiated (T1–T2, N0, M0, PSA level less than 20, Grade Group 2). • **Stage IIC:** The tumour is found only inside the prostate, and it may be large enough to be felt during DRE. The PSA level is medium. The cancer cells may be moderately or poorly differentiated (T1–T2, N0, M0, PSA level is less than 20, Grade Group 3–4).

(Continued)

Table 19.1 (Continued)

Clinical/Pathological Tumour Staging	Cancer Stage Grouping
T3: The tumour has grown through the prostate on 1 side and into the tissue just outside the prostate.	**Stage III:** PSA levels are high, the tumour is growing, or the cancer is high grade. These all indicate a locally advanced cancer that is likely to grow and spread.
• **T3a:** The tumour has grown through the prostate either on 1 or both sides of the prostate. This called extra prostatic extension (EPE).	• **Stage IIIA:** The cancer has spread beyond the outer layer of the prostate into nearby tissues. It may also have spread to the seminal vesicles. The PSA level is high. (T1–T2, N0, M0, PSA level is 20 or more, Grade Group 1–4).
• **T3b:** The tumour has grown into the seminal vesicle(s), the tube(s) that carry semen.	• **Stage IIIB:** The tumour has grown outside of the prostate gland and may have invaded nearby structures, such as the bladder or rectum (T3–T4, N0, M0, any PSA, Grade Group 1–4).
	• **Stage IIIC:** The cancer cells across the tumour are poorly differentiated, meaning they look very different from healthy cells (any T, N0, M0, any PSA, Grade Group 5).
T4: The tumour is fixed, or it is growing into nearby structures other than the seminal vesicles, such as the external sphincter, the part of the muscle layer that helps to control urination; the rectum; the bladder; levator muscles; or the pelvic wall.	**Stage IV:** The cancer has spread beyond the prostate.
	• **Stage IVA:** The cancer has spread to the regional lymph nodes (any T, N1, M0, any PSA, any Grade Group).
	• **Stage IVB:** The cancer has spread to distant lymph nodes, other parts of the body, or to the bones (any T, N0, M1, any PSA, any Grade Group).

Source: AJCC Cancer Staging Manual, 8th Edition © 2017 Springer Nature.

approach. Clearly MRI also has the ability to assess pelvic lymph nodes, and bone metastases in the imaged skeleton.

Bone scan/single photo emission computed tomography (SPECT) radionucleotide scans, or bone scintigraphy, are nuclear medicine scans to assess the whole skeleton. Patients should be warned to expect a number of hours wait between attending for an injection of radionucleotide tracer and returning for the scan itself which takes 30–60 minutes. The radioisotope technetium-99 is taken up by metabolically active bone, including areas of sclerotic bone metastases. Previous trauma, or rheumatological conditions can lead to false positives. Some centres combine CT with bone scans, to allow for three-dimensional interpretation – known as 'single photo emission computed tomography' (SPECT).

CT of the chest, abdomen and pelvis is used to stage for nodal and distant metastases.

Prostate specific membrane antigen (PSMA) positron emission tomography (PET) is starting to translate into clinical practice not only in the assessment of biochemical recurrence (PSA rise >0.02 after radical treatment) but also for primary staging and treatment planning.

Biopsy

Biopsy of the prostate should be 'influenced' by MRI findings. This may mean a 'cognitive' biopsy, whereby the clinician targets the suspicious area, or a targeted biopsy using a fusion technique combining real-time trans-rectal ultrasound with the MRI-defined target. It is routine practice to combine an approach of targeted biopsy with systematic biopsy – of non-suspicious areas. However, the multi-centre PRECISION study suggested that omitting systematic biopsy would reduce the number of low-risk diagnoses without significantly reducing detection of clinically significant disease.

Techniques

Trans-rectal biopsy is effective for targeting most of the peripheral zone, but is associated with infection and sepsis in up to 5% of patients, some of whom will require hospitalisation. The apex, and lesions in very large prostates can also be difficult to reach. Trans-perineal (TP) biopsies are safer because the biopsy needle traverses the perineum, which can be sterilised and has potential advantages in accessing the whole prostate. Traditionally TP biopsies required general anaesthesia, and often employed a 'template' grid placed in front of the perineum. 'Mapping' biopsies or 'saturation' biopsies used numerous biopsies (up to 48) to sample most of the prostate, but should no longer be used in initial assessment. However, increasingly, TP biopsies can be performed under local anaesthesia (LA), either by employing LA blocks, or by using TP access systems such as 'Precision Point' to minimise the amount of LA required and maintain an ambulatory service. Most biopsy protocols include 2–4 cores from each target and between 12 and 24 systematic cores.

Risk Categorisation

Localised prostate cancer is generally differentiated into low, intermediate, and high-risk according to derivations of the D'Amico classification (Table 19.2). Some stratification criteria further divide groups into based upon GS 7 differences (GS 3 + 4 vs GS 4 + 3) or biopsy characteristics.

Table 19.2 National Institute for Health and Care Excellence (NICE) risk classification.

Level of risk	PSA		Gleason score		Clinical stage
Low risk	< 10 ng/ml	and	≤6	and	T1 toT2a
Intermediate risk	10–20 ng/ml	or	7	or	T2b
High risk	>20 ng/ml	or	8–10	or	2≥T2c

Treatment

Non-metastatic Disease

Prostate cancer treatment decisions rely upon adequate staging of the disease and thorough counselling of the patient. Treatment options include active surveillance (AS), radical prostatectomy (open, laparoscopic, or robotic, which is by far the most common approach), external beam radiotherapy, and brachytherapy. 'All options' may be reasonable for low and intermediate-risk disease, AS should not be recommended for high-risk disease. Brachytherapy is rarely offered to patients with significant LUTS or a very large prostate gland. No superiority of one treatment against another has been demonstrated in randomised controlled trials (Hamdy et al. 2016) such that decision-making is often driven by patient perceptions towards treatment side effects and burden. It is good practice for patients to meet with oncologists and surgeons in making their decision. Radiotherapy is more effective following a time on androgen deprivation therapy. Androgen deprivation monotherapy is a potential option for men unfit for other treatment. Focal therapies such as High intensity focused ultrasound (HIFU) or cryotherapy are available at some centres – long term outcome data are awaited.

The predominant side effects of treatment are urinary symptoms, sexual dysfunction and bowel dysfunction. Radiotherapy has higher rates of bowel dysfunction, whereas surgery has higher rates of impotence or incontinence. However, side-effect outcomes from all treatments are improving with modern surgical techniques (including robotic approaches) and better targeting. Individual decision aids are advised for use with patients, one example is the Predict Prostate tool (http://prostate.predict.nhs.uk).

Advanced or Metastatic Disease

Management of advanced disease is predominantly led by oncologists, with androgen deprivation therapy remaining the workhorse of treatment. In recent years, numerous new chemotherapeutic and hormonal treatments (including docetaxel, enzalutamide, abiraterone) have been added to the armoury of oncologists, with strong evidence of beneficial effect. Novel bone-targeting therapies and increasing use of focused radiotherapy, such as radium-223 and stereotactic ablative radiotherapy (SABR), respectively, have provided improved outcomes even in advanced disease. Newly diagnosed men starting on androgen blockade should be commenced on an anti-androgen (e.g., bicalutamide) if a luteinizing hormone-releasing hormone (LHRH) agonist (e.g., goserelin acetate) is to be used for medical castration. This avoids the potential risk of 'tumour-flare' related to starting on an LHRH agonist. LHRH agonists (e.g. Degarelix) or surgical castration are other rapid mechanisms for androgen blockade.

Key Points

1) PSA is an imprecise tool. Be aware of causes of false positives.
2) Prostate cancer will often be completely asymptomatic
3) mpMRI is invaluable before prostate biopsy in men likely to be suitable for radical treatments.
4) Clinicians should move towards using the more intuitive 1–5 Grade Group system.
5) Treatment decision-making in localised disease is often complex, requiring good patient counselling via a multi-disciplinary approach.
6) Treatment options available for advanced disease continue to improve.

Further Reading

Drost, F.J.H., Osses, D.F., Nieboer, D. et al. (2019). Prostate MRI, with or without MRI-targeted biopsy, and systematic biopsy for detecting prostate cancer. *Cochrane Database of Systematic Reviews*: CD012663.

Hamdy, F.C., Donovan, J.L., Lane, J.A. et al. (2016). 10-year outcomes after monitoring, surgery, or radiotherapy for localized prostate cancer. (The ProtecT trial). *New England Journal of Medicine* 375: 1415–1424.

Kasivisvanthan, V., Rannikko, A.S., Borghi, M. et al. (2018). MRI-targeted or standard biopsy for prostate cancer diagnosis. *New England Journal of Medicine* 378: 1767–1777.

Mottet, N., Cornford, P., van den Bergh, R.C.N. et al. (2018). Prostate Cancer. European Association of Urology. http://uroweb.org/guideline/prostate-cancer.

Meyer, A.R., Joice, G.A., Schwen, Z.R. et al. (2018). Initial experience performing in-office ultrasound-guided transperineal prostate biopsy under local anaesthetic using the precision point trans perineal access system. *Urology* 115: 8–13.

20

Renal Cancer

Diagnosis and Management in the Outpatient Clinic

Karan Wadhwa

With the rise in use of cross-sectional imaging, renal masses are increasingly being diagnosed and present a common referral to the urologist both acutely and on an outpatient basis. This chapter will present a brief overview of the diagnosis and provide guidance on the management of renal masses.

Incidence

Renal cancer makes up 2–3% of all cancer diagnoses with an increase in 2% over the past 20 years. 40% are diagnosed at a late stage, and renal cancer accounts for 3% of all cancer deaths, however kidney cancer survival overall has increased over the last 40 years. Men are more likely to be diagnosed than women (1.5 : 1), with a peak incidence between the ages of 60–70 and more likely in white races than Asians or black races.

Aetiology

The main risk factors for developing renal cancer appear to be hypertension, smoking, and obesity. The genomic changes for the development of renal cancer start in childhood or adolescence and there is an increased risk with an affected first-degree relative. Several genetic conditions also predispose to renal cancer such as Von-Hippel Lindau disease, but only 8–10% of renal cancers are hereditary.

Ambulatory Urology and Urogynaecology, First Edition. Edited by Abhay Rane and Ajay Rane.
© 2021 John Wiley & Sons Ltd. Published 2021 by John Wiley & Sons Ltd.

Subtypes

The most common histological subtype of renal cancer is clear cell renal cell carcinoma (ccRCC), which also has the worst overall survival compared to papillary or chromophobe cancers. Papillary type renal cancer can be divided into type 1 and type 2 with distinct genetic features but overall with a higher survival rate than ccRCC. Lastly, chromophobe renal cancer has a myriad of genetic changes but has the best recurrence free and overall survival of the three main subtypes (see Table 20.1). Several other subtypes exist, but these make up only 10–15% of renal cancers and have variable clinical courses.

Signs and Symptoms

Onset of renal cancer is usually insidious, and over half of renal cancers are diagnosed incidentally. The classic triad of loin pain, palpable flank mass, and visible haematuria is fortunately rare (6–8%) and usually indicates a poor prognosis. Up to one-third of patients may suffer a paraneoplastic syndrome for example deranged LFTS (Stauffer's syndrome). Breathlessness or cough may indicate lung metastases or pulmonary emboli and likewise back pain may indicate a metastatic process.

Abdominal signs are usually absent, but one must be mindful to examine for chest/abdominal lymphadenopathy, a flank mass, or a varicocele (particularly right-sided).

Investigation

Alongside clinical examination, urine should be dipped for haematuria, and baseline bloods including full blood count, urea, and electrolytes, liver function tests, bone profile, and lactate dehydrogenase should be measured in clinic. Aside from clinically diagnosed tumours, the patient usually comes to hospital with imaging

Table 20.1 Subtypes of renal cancer.

Cancer-specific survival	5 years (%)	10 years (%)	15 years (%)	20 years (%)
Clear-cell RCC	71 (69–73)	62 (60–64)	56 (53–58)	52 (49–55)
Papillary RCC	91 (88–94)	86 (82–89)	85 (81–89)	83 (78–88)
Chromophobe RCC	88 (83–94)	86 (80–92)	84 (77–91)	81 (72–90)

Source: Adapted from EAU guidelines (Ljungberg et al. 2018).

such as an abdominal/renal ultrasound or CT scan. To accurately stage a patient with suspected renal cancer, a dedicated CT of chest, abdomen, and pelvis should be performed with contrast. The key features of a renal mass are size, location, enhancement (>20–30 Hounsfield units), invasion e.g. renal vein/IVC or adrenal, lymph node status, and metastases (lung/liver/bone). It is also important to consider the contralateral kidney in terms of presence, size, and shape.

In case of any diagnostic doubts, or if the patient has poor renal function, an MRI can be considered. Magnetic imaging resonance can also be used for operative planning in the case of inferior vena cava (IVC) thrombus, to assess extent of invasion and the need to mobilise the liver if the caval tumour thrombus encroaches the hepatic veins.

Dimercaptosuccinic acid (DMSA) may be useful in the case of a small contralateral kidney or if the patient has poor renal function to predict the need for peri or post-operative renal replacement therapy.

Staging

Staging is performed using the TNM (tumour location, lymph node involvement, metastatic spread) classification.

2017 TNM classification system

T – Primary tumour		
TX	Primary tumour cannot be assessed	
T0	No evidence of primary tumour	
T1	Tumour <7 cm or less in greatest dimension, limited to the kidney	
	T1a	Tumour <4 cm or less
	T1b	Tumour >4 cm but <7 cm
T2	Tumour >7 cm in greatest dimension, limited to the kidney	
	T2a	Tumour >7 cm but <10 cm
	T2b	Tumours >10 cm, limited to the kidney
T3	Tumour extends into major veins or perinephric tissues but not into the ipsilateral adrenal gland and not beyond Gerota fascia	

(Continued)

(Continued)

T3a		Tumour grossly extends into the renal vein or its segmental (muscle-containing) branches, or tumour invades perirenal and/or renal sinus fat (peripelvic fat), but not beyond Gerota fascia
T3b		Tumour grossly extends into the vena cava below diaphragm
T3c		Tumour grossly extends into vena cava above the diaphragm or invades the wall of the vena cava
T4	Tumour invades beyond Gerota fascia (including contiguous extension into the ipsilateral adrenal gland)	
N – Regional lymph nodes		
NX	Regional lymph nodes cannot be assessed	
N0	No regional lymph node metastasis	
N1	Metastasis in regional lymph node(s)	
M – Distant metastasis		
M0	No distant metastasis	
M1	Distant metastasis	

Role of Biopsy

The role of biopsy for renal cancer has been controversial in the past; however, it has recently seen a resurgence and can be safely performed as an ambulatory procedure. Biopsy is mainly indicated for those in whom we are considering active surveillance, ablative therapy, or if there is diagnostic uncertainty in the context of metastatic disease. Cystic masses are not ideal for biopsy. Concordance between biopsy histology and final specimen pathology is greater than 95%, and with the coaxial approach, biopsy yield is high. Although biopsy is generally a safe procedure, it does carry with it the risk of bleeding (4%) but clinically significant haemorrhage is rare. Biopsy tract seeding, although described, is very rare.

Management

The management of renal masses can be divided into small renal mass (T1), renal mass (T2), or metastatic RCC (mRCC). The multidisciplinary team comprising radiology, pathology, and urology renal cancer surgeons are vital in the decision-making process, taking into account patient, tumour, and resource factors.

Studies have shown no difference in cancer specific outcomes between radical and partial nephrectomy, and preservation of GFR has been shown to increase overall survival (Go et al. 2004), but studies have yet to prove an overall survival benefit from partial nephrectomy. Despite this, many authors propose doing a partial nephrectomy when possible, especially for a T1 mass. However, active surveillance is a valuable option, particularly for the more elderly or co-morbid patient. Progression on active surveillance to metastatic disease is rare (1%), and tumours are generally slow growing. Minimally invasive treatment such as renal radiofrequency ablation or cryotherapy may have a role in management of the small renal mass. Treatment such as RFA or cryotherapy may be indicated in the unfit or elderly patient, by patient choice, or for example, if there is radiological or clinical progression whilst on surveillance in a patient who does not want surgery.

Laparoscopic radical nephrectomy is the accepted standard of care for the >T1 renal mass and it is widely performed. The ipsilateral adrenal gland or lymph nodes are not routinely taken, unless there is clinical indication such as radiological extension. Open nephrectomy is now reserved for the very large renal mass, or if renal vein/IVC thrombus is suspected.

In the unfit patient with haematuria or flank pain, embolization of the tumour may be deployed in a palliative setting.

In the context of mRCC, systemic therapy such as tyrosine kinase inhibitors are generally preferred if the disease burden outside of the kidney is high. Newer agents such as the Programmed death-ligand 1 (PDL1) inhibitor Nivolumab have shown promise in clinical trials. Cytoreductive nephrectomy is reserved for palliation but may still have a role, for example, in those with low volume metastatic disease with a good performance status and favourable risk scores (Memorial Sloan Kettering Cancer Center/International Metastatic RCC Database Consortium [MSKCC/IMDC] <4). Evidence for surgical management of mRCC is poor as trials are difficult to run and recruit to.

Enhanced Recovery After Renal Surgery

Laparoscopic/robotic partial or radical nephrectomy is an operation conducive for short stay surgery. Many patients can be discharged the next post-operative day. This relies on a motivated, appropriately counselled patient and functional enhanced recovery programme. Techniques such as catheter-less nephrectomy, mobilising the patient very early the next post-operative day and consultant-review-driven discharge can reduce length of stay.

Further Reading

Go, A.S., Chertow, G.M., Fan, D. et al. (2004). Chronic kidney disease and the risks of death, cardiovascular events, and hospitalization. *New England Journal of Medicine* 351: 1296–1305. https://doi.org/10.1056/NEJMoa041031.

Ljungberg, B., Albiges, L., Bensalah, K. et al. (2019). Renal cell carcinoma. European Association of Urology. http://uroweb.org/guideline/renal-cell-carcinoma.

21

Penile Cancer

Diagnosis and Management in the Outpatient Clinic

Karen Randhawa and Hussain Alnajjar

Penile cancer is a rare disease (<1 per 100000 men) that constitutes 0.2% of all male malignancies with the most common age of presentation in the sixth decade. Early diagnosis is key as the disease can result in devastating disfigurement and a five-year survival rate of approximately 50%.It can be cured in over 80% of cases if diagnosed early and hence the need for thorough assessment and prompt treatment. There is clear evidence that centralisation of penile cancer care in the UK has led to improved outcomes; as a result, a number of other countries have followed the UK model.

Pathology

Over 95% are subtypes of squamous cell carcinoma most commonly arising from the inner prepuce or glans penis.

Risk Factors

Presence of a phimotic foreskin/chronic inflammation. Phimosis is strongly associated with invasive penile cancer.

Penile cancer is rarely seen in populations where neonatal or childhood circumcision is routinely performed. The protective effect is probably due to a decreased risk of human papilloma virus (HPV) infection in addition to reduced risk of phimosis and chronic inflammation.

Human papilloma virus: HPV types 16 and 18 are associated with approximately 45–80% of penile cancers. HPV DNA has been identified in 70–100% of intra-epithelial neoplasia and in 30–40% of invasive penile cancer.

Ambulatory Urology and Urogynaecology, First Edition. Edited by Abhay Rane and Ajay Rane.
© 2021 John Wiley & Sons Ltd. Published 2021 by John Wiley & Sons Ltd.

Lichen sclerosus: The incidence of lichen sclerosus is relatively high in penile cancer but is not associated with adverse histopathological features, including penile intraepithelial neoplasia (PeIN).

Smoking/tobacco use: The risk of penile cancer is increased fivefold in smokers versus non-smokers. Similarly chewing tobacco is a significant risk factor.

Exposure to ultraviolet radiation: Psoriasis patients undergoing psoralen plus ultraviolet A (PUVA) treatment have an increased penile cancer incidence of 286 times compared to the general population. Patients treated for psoriasis with immunosuppressive drugs also appear to have an increased risk of developing penile cancer.

Human immunodeficiency viruses (HIV) infection: There is reported to be an eightfold increased risk of penile cancer in patients with HIV.

Multiple sexual partners/early age of first intercourse: Evidence suggests that there is a three- to fivefold increased risk of penile cancer associated with multiple sexual partners.

Other epidemiological risk factors are low socioeconomic status and a low level of education.

Presentation

Pre-malignant lesions and benign penile dermatoses may present as a rash, small red lesions or raised area on the penis. It is important that clinicians are aware of the need for biopsy and a prompt referral on to a specialist centre where appropriate.

Patients may also present with phimosis, making it difficult to visualise the lesion, in addition to penile pain, palpable lesion, problems voiding, foul odour, bleeding, or discharge from the penis.

Presentation can also be late, with obvious fungating penile lesions and/or metastatic groin node masses.

History

It is important to assess the overall health of the patient in terms of co-morbidities including past medical and surgical history.

Ask specific questions relating to:

- Location and size of the lesion
- Duration
- Is the lesion growing?

- Previous similar lesions?
- Any voiding symptoms?
- Associated pain
- Bleeding/Discharge?
- Any problems retracting the foreskin?
- Previous surgery to penis/foreskin
- Sexual history – sexually active?

Examination

General examination should be performed to assess the overall health of the patient.

Primary Lesion (May Be Hidden Under Phimosis)

If it is possible to retract the foreskin, perform a visual examination of the glans assessing the size, location, and morphology of any glans lesions (exophytic or ulcerative). Proximity to the meatus should also be assessed. Palpation of the lesion, glans penis, and penile shaft should be performed to assess for corporal involvement.

Assess foreskin for lichen sclerosis, warts, scarring, change in colour, or any evidence of pre-malignant disease.

Lymph Nodes

Palpate both groins for any palpable lymph nodes. If palpable lymph nodes identified – document number, laterality and whether fixed or mobile. Oedema of the penis, scrotum, and/or legs may occur.

Investigation

Role of Penile Biopsy

In practice, for suspected inflammatory penile lesions, early biopsy is required to confirm diagnosis and exclude carcinoma, if there a is lack of early and adequate response to appropriate medical therapy. For suspicious raised lesions and obvious cancers, immediate biopsy can both confirm malignancy and offer information on cancer subtype, grade, and stage to guide further investigation and management. The procedure may be carried out under local anaesthetic penile block or general anaesthetic and may require a dorsal slit to visualise the lesion fully prior to biopsy. Lesions inside the meatus may be difficult to biopsy endoscopically and may therefore require a meatotomy to expose the lesion before performing a biopsy. In any event, this can normally be achieved as an ambulatory procedure.

Although a punch biopsy may be sufficient for superficial lesions, an excisional biopsy deep enough to properly assess the degree of invasion and stage is preferable. It is also helpful to include normal adjacent tissue to allow examination of the interface between normal tissue and tumour.

Imaging

Penis

Magnetic resonance imaging (MRI) with a pharmacologically induced (e.g., alprostadil) erection has a role in penile-preserving surgery, and it is a useful tool when assessing for corporal involvement.

Magnetic resonance imaging may also be helpful in advanced local disease to assess extent of invasion and presence of skip lesions; this can help with surgical planning pre-operatively.

Ultrasound may accurately determine the degree of corporal invasion; however, it cannot predict invasion of corpus spongiosum in smaller glans tumours.

Regional Lymph Nodes

Penile cancer demonstrates a step-wise lymphogenic spread, primarily to nodes in the inguinal region. Following this, metastasis to the pelvic nodes can then occur with subsequent haematogenic dissemination.

Cancer staging by early assessment for regional lymph node metastases is key to determining disease prognosis and appropriate lymph node management.

Impalpable Lymph Nodes

In patients with no palpable nodes, approximately 20% will have micro-metastatic disease. However, the role of CT and MRI in the nodal staging of the disease is limited when the nodes are impalpable.

European Association of Urology (EAU) guidelines state that imaging studies are not helpful in staging clinically normal inguinal regions, although they may be used in obese patients where palpation is unreliable. Further management of patients with normal inguinal nodes should be guided by pathological risk factors of the primary tumour. Lympho-vascular invasion, local stage, and grade of the primary tumour are predictive of lymphatic metastasis. Invasive lymph node staging is required in patients at intermediate or high risk of lymphatic spread.

Dynamic sentinel node biopsy (DSNB) has become established as an accurate technique for assessment of inguinal lymph node status. In experienced hands, sensitivity may be increased when combined with preoperative groin node ultrasound with fine needle aspiration cytology for nodal staging. (95% sensitivity).

Dynamic sentinel node biopsy technique involves intradermal technetium-99 m radio-isotope injection to the distal penis, followed by SPECT–CT imaging to localise the sentinel node. Identification of sentinel node/s at surgery is optimised by combined use of a gamma probe and penile intradermal patent bleu injection intraoperatively. The technique is relatively simple with low post-operative complication rate.

Alternatively, superficial modified inguinal lymphadenectomy maybe performed where medial superficial inguinal lymph nodes and those from the central zone are removed preserving the long saphenous vein. This can be performed with frozen section examination, where, if any positive lymph nodes are identified, patients proceed to radical inguinal lymphadenectomy on the ipsilateral side at the same time.

Palpable Lymph Nodes

Imaging for palpable disease by computerized tomography (CT) or MRI may be used to assess the size, extent, location, and structures that are in close proximity to the involved node, as well as the presence of pelvic and retroperitoneal lymph nodes and distant metastasis.

Distant Metastases

The presence of metastatic pelvic lymph nodes is associated with a poor prognosis in penile cancer patients. Therefore, CT staging is often in practice carried out pre-operatively.

The EAU guidelines advocate staging for systemic metastases in patients with positive inguinal nodes. Abdominal and pelvic CT is recommended in addition to a chest X-ray or thoracic CT. Positron emission tomography/CT (PET/CT) is also an option with a diagnostic accuracy of 96%.

Management

Management options are determined by the stage of disease taken in conjunction with patient factors such as age, comorbidities, and performance status.

Management of the Primary Lesion

The aims of treatment of the primary tumour are complete tumour removal with as much organ preservation as possible and without compromising oncological control. A clearance of 3–5 mm from the surgical margin is deemed adequate. Local recurrences have been shown to have little influence on long-term survival justifying the adoption of organ preservation strategies in order to minimise the disfiguring effects of the surgery and its devastating psychological effects.

Treatment options are determined principally by the site of the lesion and degree of invasion.

Superficial Non-invasive Disease

Even in the absence of foreskin involvement, circumcision should be performed to facilitate treatment, surveillance, and reduce potential recurrence. Other treatment options are:

Topical chemotherapy with imiquimod or 5-FU can be offered. This is an outpatient self-applied treatment. Significant and uncomfortable inflammatory response can occur to treatment. Complete response rates of 57% are reported.

Laser treatment with Nd: YAG or CO2 laser. This can be performed under local or short general anaesthetic as a day-case procedure; however, it is not routinely used.

Partial or Total Glans Resurfacing

This involves excision of part or all of the glans epithelium and subepithelial layer with application of a split skin graft under general anaesthesia. It is an effective primary treatment or following failure of topical/laser therapy.

Invasive Disease

Disease confined to the foreskin can be dealt with by circumcision alone providing that negative surgical margins can be achieved. Small invasive glans lesions can be treated effectively by partial glansectomy and glans reconstruction for optimal functional results. Larger lesions (>T2) necessitates total glansectomy with or without extra-genital split skin graft reconstruction to the corporal heads.

Lesions invading the distal corpora are typically managed with partial penectomy with good cosmetic results by split skin graft application to the repaired corporal bodies.

For the majority of lesions invading corpora, either standard partial or total penectomy with perineal urethrostomy is appropriate, the choice depending on whether a useful functional penile length can be achieved by partial penectomy.

Most surgery for primary penile cancer is feasible as ambulatory day-case or overnight-stay surgery, depending largely on social and home circumstances. Traditionally postoperative care of procedures involving split-skin grafting dictated a longer inpatient stay; however, secure fixation of the penile graft dressings using sutures tied over the dressing can allow early mobilisation and completion of care as ambulatory surgery.

Lymph Node Management

Early treatment of inguinal node disease is a critical factor influencing prognosis. Patients with clinically positive nodes and those with positive fine needle aspiration cytology (FNAC) or positive sentinel node biopsy require a radical inguinal node dissection on the affected side. Open radical inguinal node dissection carries a significant risk of post-operative complications, reported in up to 55% in some studies often resulting in prolonged inpatient care.

Minimally invasive video-endoscopic inguinal lymphadenectomy (VEIL) has been developed using laparoscopic/robotic-assisted techniques to reduce associated morbidity and hospital stay for patients with small-volume nodal disease. Reported series have shown 20% overall morbidity with significantly reduced rates of wound problems and lymphoedema.

Ipsilateral iliac node dissection is indicated when two or more nodes are involved or where there is extracapsular nodal disease on histopathology of the sentinel node. Laparoscopic iliac node dissection reduces post-operative recovery time and reduces hospital stay.

Adjuvant chemotherapy has been shown to improve survival for patients with stage N2/N3 disease.

Follow-Up after Treatment

The aim of follow-up is the early detection of both local and regional nodal recurrence. Both occur most commonly within two years and are rare after five years. Outpatient assessment and surveillance of penile cancer patients is by physical examination of the penis and groins. Groin ultrasound ± FNAC can be used as an adjunct to physical examination for early detection of regional node recurrence. Table 21.1 summarises the follow-up protocol adopted from EAU guidelines (Hakenberg et al. 2019).

Table 21.1 Guidelines for follow-up in penile cancer.

	Interval of follow-up		Examinations and Investigations	Minimum duration of follow-up	Strength rating
	Years one to two	**Years three to five**			
Recommendations for follow-up of the primary tumour					
Penile-preserving treatment	Three months	Six months	Regular physician or self-examination. Repeat biopsy after topical or laser treatment for penile intraepithelial neoplasia.	Five years	Strong
Amputation	Three months	One year	Regular physician or self-examination.	Five years	Strong
Recommendations for follow-up of the inguinal lymph nodes					
Surveillance	Three months	Six months	Regular physician or self-examination.	Five years	Strong
pN0 at Initial treatment	Three months	One year	Regular physician or self-examination. Ultrasound with fine-needle aspiration biopsy optional.	Five years	Strong
pN+ at initial treatment	Three months	Six months	Regular physician or self-examination. Ultrasound with fine-needle aspiration cytology optional, computed tomography/magnetic resonance Imaging optional.	Five years	Strong

Source: From EAU guidelines on Penile Cell © 2017 Uroweb.

Summary of Key Points

- Have a high index of suspicion for penile lesions and arrange prompt biopsy to confirm diagnosis.
- Accurate local staging with physical examination, biopsy, and MRI can guide appropriate penile-sparing surgical treatment to optimise functional and cosmetic outcomes.
- Early invasive inguinal node assessment with DSNB can allow appropriate staging and early treatment for inguinal node metastases whilst minimising morbidity from unnecessary negative inguinal node dissection.
- The early detection and treatment of inguinal node metastases is vital to improve chances of survival.

Further Reading

Alnajjar, H.M., Lam, W., Bolgeri, M. et al. (2012). Treatment of carcinoma in situ of the glans penis with topical chemotherapy agents. *Eur. Urol.* 62: 923.

Barocas, D. and Chang, S. (2010). Penile cancer: clinical presentation, diagnosis, and staging. *Urol. Clin. North Am.* 37 (3): 343–352.

Bloom, J.B., Stern, M., Patel, N.H. et al. (2018). Detection of lymph node metastases in penile cancer. *Transl. Androl. Urol.* 7 (5): 879–886.

Clark, P.E., Spiess, P.E., Agarwal, N. et al. (2013). Penile cancer: clinical practice guidelines in oncology. *J. Natl. Compr. Canc. Netw.* 11 (5): 594–615.

Hakenberg, O.W., Compérat, E., Minhas, S. et al. (2019). Penile Cancer. European Association of Urology. http://uroweb.org/guideline/penile-cancer.

Sharma, P., Djajadiningrat, R., Zargar-Shoshtari, K. et al. (2015). Adjuvant chemotherapy is associated with improved overall survival in pelvic node-positive penile cancer after lymph node dissection: a multi-institutional study. *Urol. Oncol.* 33: 496 e17.

22

Testis Cancer

Diagnosis and Management in the Outpatient Clinic

Benjamin Patel

Testicular cancer (TC) is the most common solid cancer in men aged 20–45 with around 2400 new cases in 2016 in the UK. It constitutes 1% of male cancers and 5% of urological tumours. Since the early 1990s, the incidence has increased by 28% in males in the UK. The incidence is projected to further rise by 12% in the UK between 2015 and 2035 to 10/10000 males. There is a peak incidence between 30 and 34 and it is rarely found in those below 15 years and above 60 years. (See Figure 22.1.) Encouragingly, mortality has fallen since the introduction of platinum-based chemotherapy, with a 98% 10-year survival in the UK. Indeed, in 2016 there were less than 60 deaths.

Aetiology

Aetiological factors are largely non-modifiable. TC is more common in white western Caucasians. The most commonly affected age group is 20–45 years and there is a variable histological pattern of disease according to age. Non-seminomatous germ cell tumours (NSGCTs) affect a slightly younger cohort (20–35 years) compared to seminomas (35–45 years). Infants and children below 10 years most commonly develop yolk sac tumours and 50% of TCs in those >60 years are lymphoma.

A previous diagnosis of TC is associated with a 12-fold increased risk of metachronous TC, with bilateral TCs occurring in 1–2% of cases. 5–10% of TC patients have a history of cryptorchidism. In unilateral cryptorchidism, TC risk is 6 times greater in the undescended testicle and 1.7 times increased in the descended testicle. One large study indicated that those who undergo early orchidopexy (<13 years) have a twofold increased risk of TC, compared to a fivefold increased risk in those undergoing late orchidopexy (>13 years).

Ambulatory Urology and Urogynaecology, First Edition. Edited by Abhay Rane and Ajay Rane.

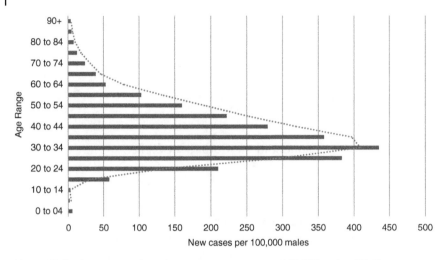

Figure 22.1 Average number of new cases per year per 100,000 males, UK. *Source:* Based on graphic created by Cancer Research UK.

Genetic factors have also been identified. TC is 5 times higher in men with an affected father and 8–9 times higher in men with an affected brother. Additionally, Kleinfelter's syndrome and Kallman's syndrome are associated with increased TC risk.

In general, TC is not clearly linked to preventable factors. Human immunodeficiency virus HIV appears to increase risk of TC by 30–40%. There is weak evidence for chemical carcinogens and rural residence increasing risk. However, there is no strong evidence for smoking, alcohol, vasectomy, or trauma increasing risk.

Finally, Testicular carcinoma in situ, also known as intratubular germ cell neoplasia (ITGCN) or testicular intraepithelial neoplasia (TIN), is a precursor for TC; around 50% of men with cancer in situ (CIS) will develop TC within five years without treatment.

Symptoms and Signs

Testicular cancer most commonly presents as a hard, painless lump. It is slightly more common on the right side and bilateral in 1–2% of cases. Five percent of TCs present with acute scrotal pain, secondary to intra-tumoral haemorrhage. Ten percent unfortunately present with symptoms of advanced disease, including weight loss, lumps in the neck, bone pain, chest symptoms and neurological symptoms. Lumbar back pain may occur if the psoas muscles and nerve roots are affected.

A proportion of TCs present during routine clinical examination, casual ultrasound (US) findings, or are revealed by scrotal trauma. On examination by bimanual palpation, testicular asymmetry may be identified. A hard, non-tender, irregular and non-trans illuminable mass may be felt in the testis. An associated hydrocele may be present if the tunica albuginea is breached. The epididymis, spermatic cord, and scrotal wall may be normal or involved in a small proportion of cases. Endocrine manifestations of certain TCs may results in gynaecomastia. Metastatic disease may result in supraclavicular lymphadenopathy, abdominal masses, hepatomegaly, lower limb oedema, chest signs, and cachexia.

Pathology and Subtypes

The majority of TCs are germ cell tumours (GCTs), subcategorised into seminomatous germ cell tumour (SGCT) and non-seminomatous germ cell tumour (NSGCT) (see Table 22.1). Classic seminomas are well circumscribed, homogenous firm pale tumours. Anaplastic seminomas are similar to classic seminomas but have increased numbers of mitoses. Spermatocytic seminomas are found in an older cohort of men and are generally benign. Teratomas are heterogenous tumours composed of elements of fully differentiated tissue: mesoderm (bone, cartilage, muscle), ectoderm (neural tissue and stratified squamous including skin and derivatives such as hair follicles) and endoderm (including mucus glands).

Investigation

Ultrasound (US) is the first line investigation of scrotal lumps, with a sensitivity of almost 100% and will confirm whether a lump is intra- or extra testicular. It is inexpensive and should be performed to explore the abnormal and contralateral testes. Magnetic resonance imaging (MRI) of the scrotum has a greater sensitivity and specificity than US in diagnosing TC, but its high cost obviates its routine use.

Serum tumour markers play a role in diagnosis and differentiation, and they also have a prognosticating role. Alpha-fetaprotein (AFP) (produced by yolk sac cells), human chorionic gonadotropin (hCG) (produced by trophoblasts) and lactate dehydrogenase (LDH) should all be measured before and seven days after orchidectomy. Beta-hCG is elevated in 100% of choriocarcinomas, 40% of teratomas, and 10% of pure seminomas. Alpha-fetaprotein can be elevated by embryonal carcinoma, teratoma, and yolk sac tumours. Pure seminomas and choriocarcinomas are not associated with raised AFP. Lactate dehydrogenase is elevated in half of TCs and is used to assess tumour burden. It is the only elevated

Table 22.1 Testicular cancer classification and distribution.

Germ cell tumours (90–95%)	Other tumours (5–10%)
Seminoma (60%)	Stromal:
• Spermatocytic	• Leydig
• Classical	• Sertoli
• Anaplastic	• Gonadoblastoma
Non-seminomatous (40%)	Lymphoma
• Teratoma (mature, immature)	Metastatic from other site (<1%)
• Yolk sac tumour	Rhabdomyosarcoma
• Embryonal	Adenomatoid tumour
• Choriocarcinoma	Epidermoid cyst (benign)
• Mixed	

marker in 10% of non-seminomas. PLAP is elevated in 40% of patients with advanced germ cell tumours (GCTs), but is non-specific and falsely elevated in smokers.

Imaging plays an important role. Computerized tomography (CT) is generally undertaken of the abdomen and pelvis to analyse extra-testicular metastasis and lymph node involvement. Chest X-ray (CXR) is utilised to exclude pulmonary disease, with further imaging of chest, brain, spine, and bones where clinically indicated. Importantly, biopsy is not generally advised for the evaluation of testicular masses. Diagnosis is instead established by histological analysis of the testis after removal.

All patients with suspected testicular mass should undergo inguinal exploration, alongside exteriorisation of the testis within its tunics. If a malignant tumour is identified, orchidectomy and division of the spermatic cord at the internal inguinal ring should be carried out. This is routinely performed in the ambulatory setting.

Staging of TC includes the anatomical extent of the primary tumour (pT), regional nodes (N) and distant metastases (M), alongside the assessment of serum tumour markers after orchidectomy (S).

Management of Seminomatous Germ Cell Tumours (SGCTs)

Stage I non-locally invasive disease can be managed with surveillance, with a relapse rate of 15–20% at five years. In low-risk groups (tumour size <4 cm and no rete testis invasion), the recurrence rate may be much lower. Chemotherapy may be utilised in the case of relapse under surveillance, although the majority of patients are suitable for radiotherapy alone because of the small volume of disease at the time of recurrence. Alternatively, stage I non-locally invasive seminomas can be managed with single agent carboplatin chemotherapy. Whilst seminoma cells are extremely radiosensitive, the increased risk of radiation-induced secondary non-germ cell malignancies means that adjuvant radiotherapy is rarely used in stage I disease and has no role in young patients <40 years. Retroperitoneal lymph node dissection (RPLND) is not recommended in stage I seminoma.

Stage IIA/B seminomas may be managed with radiotherapy, with reported relapse rates of 9–24%, although long-term radiotherapy-associated morbidity such as secondary malignancies and cardiovascular events are a concern. Chemotherapy is an alternative, with similar reported relapse rates. Three cycles of bleomycin, etoposide, and cisplatin ('BEP') chemotherapy are generally employed, with four cycles of EP in cases where bleomycin toxicity is a concern.

Management of Non-seminomatous Germ Cell Tumours (NSGCTs)

Options for stage I patients include active surveillance, adjuvant chemotherapy, and RPLND. Patients should be informed about all options, including recurrence rates and potential side effects, and the ultimate decision should take into account, risk based on vascular invasion. The largest studies of surveillance strategies suggest a cumulative relapse rate of 30%. Alternatively, patients may receive adjuvant chemotherapy with BEP, which appears to reduce relapse to under 5% with minimal long-term toxicity. Salvage treatment of patients with recurrence during surveillance generally consists of three to four courses of BEP chemotherapy, followed by RPLND if necessary. The role of primary RPLND has now diminished in stage I disease, in view of the high cancer-specific survival rates of surveillance with salvage treatment and the low relapse rates if adjuvant chemotherapy is employed.

In stage IIA/B NSGCTs, chemotherapy is generally employed, except for stage II disease without elevated tumour markers, in which RPLND or surveillance can be undertaken to clarify stage of disease.

Management of Metastatic Testicular Cancer

Metastatic SGCT and NSGCT are generally managed with three cycles of chemotherapy, alongside RPLND for residual or recurrent masses and salvage chemotherapy for relapsing disease.

Further Reading

Kier, M.G., Lauritsen, J., Mortensen, M.S. et al. (2017). Prognostic factors and treatment results after bleomycin, etoposide, and cisplatin in germ cell cancer: a population-based study. *Eur. Urol.* 71: 290.

Laguna, M.P., Albers, P., Algaba, F. et al. (2019). Testicular Cancer. European Association of Urology. http://uroweb.org/guideline/testicular-cancer.

Tandstad, T., Ståhl, O., Håkansson, U. et al. (2014). One course of adjuvant BEP in clinical stage I nonseminoma mature and expanded results from the SWENOTECA group. *Ann. Oncol.* 25: 2167.

23

Plain X-Ray, Computed Tomography Scanning, and Nuclear Imaging in Urology

Tharani Mahesan

Imaging and radiological investigation are important tools in the urologist's armamentarium, and access various modalities and sound working theory for their usage is key to running an ambulatory service. Historically X-rays were the most widely used imaging modality in urology, however in recent decades computed tomography (CT) scanning is often preferred to 'plain' X-ray imaging. An X-ray is a type of transmission radiology in which an electromagnetic beam is passed through the body. Tissue- energy reactions alter the beam as it is transmitted and energy is absorbed by different tissues, to differing degrees. This varied absorption leads to production of an image at a detector or plate, but could be considered as taking a 'measurement' of those differing tissues using X-ray absorption.

Computerized tomography (CT) scanning employs an X-ray transmission source and detector that rotate about the patient, essentially taking multiple X-ray 'measurements' from multiple angles. This data is then compiled, reconstituted, and reconstructed as cross-sectional imaging.

Computerized tomography scanning allows for measurement of tissue or structure density and this is measured in Hounsfield units (HU). The higher the HU, the 'brighter' a structure appears on CT. This linear scale assigns the tissue a score relative to distilled water at standard pressure and temperature (being 0 HU) and air at standard pressure and temperature (being −1000 HU).

The Hounsfield scale is only applied to the density of tissues on medical CT scans. (See Table 23.1.)

Non-contrast CT scanning of the kidneys, ureters and bladder (so-called CT KUB) is now the gold-standard imaging modality for suspected ureteric colic. For other diagnoses, the additional use of iodinated contrast allows for further enhancement and delineation of the entire urinary tract, which can assist in identifying mass lesions, 'filling defects' or causes of ureteric obstruction. The use of intravenous contrast agents can allow some determination of the

Ambulatory Urology and Urogynaecology, First Edition. Edited by Abhay Rane and Ajay Rane.
© 2021 John Wiley & Sons Ltd. Published 2021 by John Wiley & Sons Ltd.

Table 23.1 Hounsfield values of tissues on CT scan.

Tissue	HU
Fat	−120 to −90
Bone	+1800 to 1900
Kidney	+20 to +45
Blood	+13 to +50
Blood clot	+50 to +75
Urine	−5 to +15

function of the kidney; however nuclear medicine (NM) imaging is a far superior modality for this purpose.

Clinicians need to be mindful that use of X-ray and CT is not without risk. As radiation passes through the body it is absorbed. The effect of ionising radiation on human tissues is measured in Sieverts, a derived unit that is representative of the stochastic health risk attached to the radiation. Medical scans typically have their radiation effects defined in millisieverts (mSv). It is worth noting that some tissues absorb more radiation than others. This can mean that the effective dose of radiation (whole body radiation absorbed) is higher for certain studies. (See Table 23.2.)

The ALARA (As Low As Reasonably Achievable) principle should be kept in mind when considering the necessity for use of ionising radiation for the purposes of investigation. In younger patients particularly, it should be considered whether ultrasound could reasonably answer the diagnostic question instead of an X-ray based scan. Furthermore, intravenous administration of iodinated contrast also poses its own risks – largely due to its nephrotoxicity. Patients who take metformin are at risk of developing metabolic acidosis, but this risk is dependent on level of renal function and volume of contrast given. Radiology departments will have protocols for either omitting metformin prior to or after a scan to reduce this risk. In some cases, it may be safe to continue taking metformin. Anaphylactoid reaction to injected contrast media is a rare but serious event. Previous reactions to IV contrast present a contraindication to a further contrast CT scan.

X-ray

An X-ray of the KUB can be used to look for the presence of renal or ureteric calculi. Although around 90% of renal stones are radio-opaque, most studies confirm the sensitivity of plain KUB X-ray to be around 50% for detecting stones. Due to

Table 23.2 Radiation dose (in mSv) of imaging modalities.

Type of imaging	mSv
Chest X-ray	0.02
Abdominal X-ray	0.07
IVU	3
CT KUB (low dose)	<3.5
CT KUB (ultra-low dose)	<1.9
CT abdomen and pelvis (no contrast)	10
CT abdomen and pelvis (contrast)	20
CT Urogram	15.9

the speed and simplicity of plain X-ray, however, this modality is still commonly used for re-assessment of a known stone burden or to demonstrate the passage of a known ureteric calculus.

Intravenous Pyelogram (IVP) or Intravenous Urogram (IVU)

Intravenous urogram (IVU) or intravenous pyelogram (IVP) is now becoming somewhat historic, having been supplanted by the superior sensitivity and specificity of CT for the assessment of ureteric colic. The IVU protocol consists of a pre-contrast control, followed by administration of intravenous (IV) contrast and series of plain KUB X-rays to assess the uptake of contrast into the kidneys and the excretion. The contrast delineates the shape of the kidney (nephrogram) and can demonstrate hydronephrosis and delayed drainage via a 'standing column' of contrast in a poorly draining ureter.

A single shot IVU continues to have a role in the operating theatre for 'on table' investigation of renal trauma and suspected collecting system injuries and can occasionally be useful in Shockwave Lithotripsy to help identify the location of a ureteric stone at the distal-most point of a 'standing column.'

CT KUB

CT KUB is a non-contrast, low-dose CT scan that is used most commonly for the identification of nephrolithiasis. CT KUB offers near 99% sensitivity for urinary tract calculi and allows assessment of concomitant hydronephrosis and hydroureter.

CT KUB allows for reasonable assessment of urinary tract anatomy, and for patients with a contra-indication to intravenous contrast (e.g., chronic kidney disease) it remains a useful investigation for presentations of other conditions such as haematuria and urinary tract sepsis.

CT Urogram (CTU)

CT urography is employed most commonly for the investigation of visible haematuria and involves three scan phases. A non-contrast phase (CT KUB), a further scan sequence at 60–90 seconds post-injection of contrast and a delayed scan sequence at approximately 10–15 minutes. At 60–90 seconds, the uptake of IV within the renal parenchyma produces a 'nephrographic phase.' It is in this phase that renal masses may be identified. The delayed sequence allows clinicians to visualise the drainage of the contrast from the kidney to the bladder and can identify filling defects, hydroureter, or delayed drainage.

Renal Protocol CT Scan

This scan protocol is used to characterise renal lesions. There is a pre-contrast phase followed by three further phases: the cortico-medullary phase, the nephrogenic phase, and excretory phase. The cortico-medullary phase takes place 25–40 seconds after injection of contrast. The degree of uptake of contrast within a lesion (seen as increased 'brightness') is defined as 'enhancement.' A change of greater than 20 HU is considered significant. The nephrogenic scan sequence; taken 100 seconds post contrast, allows visualisation of the vascularity of the lesion as well as presence of thrombus within the vein. As with a CT urogram (CTU), the delayed excretory phase allows delineation of the entire urinary tract and is useful in patients where transitional cell carcinoma is suspected within the collecting system.

Staging CT Scans

In patients with significant malignancy, contrast CT scans of the chest, abdomen, and pelvis are performed in order to stage the cancer. Staging is important to determine whether the disease is confined to an organ and thereby establish treatment and prognosis.

Percutaneous Procedures

Imaging guided percutaneous procedures provide an important tool in diagnostic and interventional urology. Procedures may be ultrasound, fluoroscopy, or CT guided. In most centres the renal procedures are performed by radiologists.

Renal Biopsy

Widely shunned for many years due to concerns about seeding, we are now seeing an increase in renal biopsy. Given the number of renal masses being identified incidentally, especially in younger patients, it offers the benefit of avoiding nephrectomy (partial or radical) in those that are found to benign. This is further discussed in Chapter 20, Renal Cancer.

Renal Cyst Aspiration

These are normally ultrasound guided. They are not commonly performed due to the high risk of recurrence as well as the small risk of seeding if the cyst is incorrectly characterised. All cysts must be characterised on CT using the Bosniak classification before aspiration is considered.

Aspiration and sclerosant instillation should be reserved for those who are symptomatic with very large cysts but who are not candidates for surgery either due to patient choice or fitness.

Nephrostomy and Antegrade Procedures

A nephrostomy is a drain placed percutaneously directly into the renal collecting system. It is sited by interventional radiologists under ultrasound and fluoroscopic guidance.

Common indications for nephrostomy insertion include renal obstruction secondary to malignant conditions, ureteric injuries, and impassable structuring of the ureter. Nephrostomy represents a valuable 'rescue' option where retrograde stenting has failed.

If a guide-wire can be advanced into the bladder via a nephrostomy tract, 'antegrade' ureteric stent insertion can be attempted.

Nuclear Medicine Scans

Nuclear medicine (NM) scans rely on radioactive tracers injected into the body. As the tracer decays, radiation is emitted and can be detected. This allows sensitive measurements of the quantity of tracer within the renal tract, based on the radiation emission and therefore accurate representation of renal uptake and function as well as excretion.

The most commonly used tracer isotope in urology is technetium 99, which decays to emit gamma radiation.

The use of radioactive tracers does expose the patient to a small amount of radiation that does minimally increase their cancer risk. There is a small risk of allergy to the tracer. Nuclear medicine scans are not suitable for those who are pregnant, trying for pregnancy, or breast feeding.

MAG3 Renogram

Relying on the tracer ^{99m}Tc labelled Mercapto-Acetyl Triglycine (MAG3) renograms are dynamic scans that allow for the assessment of renal uptake, processing, and excretion.

It is used to diagnose functional renal obstruction, but can also identify ureteric reflux. MAG-3 provides an estimation of split renal (right vs left) function but this is not as accurate as a dimercaptosuccinic acid (DMSA) (see next section). Perhaps the most common use is for patients with pyelo-ureteric junction obstruction (PUJO) or for assessment of outcomes in those who have undergone previous pyeloplasty.

DMSA

Like MAG 3, DMSA is labelled with ^{99m}Tc. Unlike MAG3, it is not excreted by the proximal tubules and the image obtained is a static one. By obtaining an image at three to four hours post-injection, clinicians are able to quantify the number of functioning nephrons in each kidney relative to the other side.

DMSA scans are useful for assessing split function and for monitoring for the presence of scars where nephrons may have been damaged. DMSAs may be used in patients with stag horn calculi or long standing PUJO where benign nephrectomy is being considered, or in those with renal lesions for whom a radical or partial nephrectomy is being pursued.

Bone Scan

Another static scan, bone scans are used in urology for assessment of prostatic bony metastases. Patients are injected with technetium labelled methylene diphosphonate (MDP). Methylene diphosphonate is preferentially taken up in areas with increased osteoblastic activity such as metastatic deposits.

Positron Emitting Tomography (PET)/PET CT

A positron emitting tomography (PET) scan or PET/CT scan uses radioactive tracers to identify areas of increased or altered metabolism. It is widely used in the identification and surveillance of malignancy as well as assessing response to treatment. Combining PET scans and CT scans offers both metabolic and anatomical detail. The most widely used radiotracers for PET scans in urology are 18F-fluorodeoxyglucose (FDG) and 11c-choline. These radio-isotopes decay emitting positrons, and as these travel through tissues they slow down. As they slow, they are able to interact with electrons that destroy both of them and produce gamma photons. These gamma photons are detected by a gamma camera. FDG is used in the assessment for metastases in renal and bladder cancer, as well as the staging and spread of testicular cancer. Choline PET can be used for the diagnosis, staging, and surveillance of prostate cancer.

Further Reading

Payne, S. and Eardley, I. (2012). *Imaging and Technology in Urology: Principles and Clinical Applications*. New York: Springer.

Tublin, M.E. and Nelson, J. (2018). *Imaging in Urology*. New York: Elsevier.

24

Magnetic Resonance Imaging in Urology

Benjamin Patel

In the last decade, magnetic resonance imaging (MRI) has become pivotal in the staging and investigation of urological malignancy and has had a transformative effect on prostate cancer care pathways.

Basic Principles

Nuclei, made up of protons and neutrons, are charged particles with a specific motion or 'precession.' When a human body is placed in a strong magnetic field, many of the free, randomly aligned hydrogen nuclei align themselves with the direction of the magnetic field. This behaviour is termed Larmor precession. To generate a magnetic resonance (MR) image, a radio-frequency pulse with a frequency equal to the Larmor frequency is applied perpendicular to the magnetic field, causing the net magnetic moment to tilt away from the direction of the magnetic field. Once the radio-frequency signal is halted, the nuclei realign themselves with their net magnetic moment parallel to the strong magnetic field. During this 'relaxation', the nuclei lose energy and emit their own radiofrequency signal, referred to as the 'free-induction decay (FID) response signal.' The FID response signal can then be measured by a field coil placed around the body being imaged. This measurement can be reconstructed to generate three-dimensional MR images.

There are two types of relaxation: longitudinal (T1) and transverse (T2). T1 measures the time taken for the magnetic moment of the displaced nuclei to return 63% to thermal equilibrium. Water and cerebrospinal fluid (CSF) have long T1 values, appearing dark on T1 weighted images, whereas fat has a short T1 value and appears bright. T1-weighted imaging (T1WI) is particularly useful in identifying post-biopsy haemorrhage and detecting the status of lymph nodes and skeletal

Ambulatory Urology and Urogynaecology, First Edition. Edited by Abhay Rane and Ajay Rane.

metastases, especially in combination with IV gadolinium-based contrast. T2 on the other hand measures the time required for the FID response signal to decay.

Clinical Applications

Multi-Parametric MRI in Prostate Cancer

The utility of single sequence T1WI in evaluating the prostate is limited by poor differentiation between prostate and surrounding tissues, artefact from bowel motility and poor intra-prostatic tissue resolution. Multi-parametric MRI (mpMRI) aims to obtain an ideal three-dimensional prostate image by combining T2-weighted imaging (T2WI), diffusion-weighted imaging (DWI), and dynamic contrast-enhanced imaging (DCEI). In general, intestinal motility-reducing drugs and endorectal coils are used to reduce signal artefact associated with intestinal peristalsis.

T2WI detects the low intensity of neoplastic tissue. Its high resolution provides a sharp demarcation in the prostate capsule. However, in isolation, it is poor at detecting transitional zone and central zone cancers. Diffusion-weighted imaging provides an 'apparent diffusion coefficient' (ADC) map and high b-value images. Clinically significant cancers appear hypointense in the ADC maps due to restricted diffusion. DWI is better at identifying transitional zone and central zone tumours, as well as cancer aggressiveness, but has poor resolution. DCEI uses gadolinium-based contrast agent to visualise angiogenesis and thus evaluate the vascularity of tumour.

Prostate Imaging Reporting and Data System (PI-RADS) was established in 2012 by the European Society of Urogynaecologic Radiology to standardise reporting of prostate MRI and was updated in 2015 with the release of PI-RADSV2. A score from 1 to 5 is assigned, with 1 indicating that clinically significant cancer is highly unlikely, 3 indicating that clinically significant cancer is equivocal, and 5 indicating that clinically significant cancer is highly likely. Interest in mpMRI has accelerated following publication of PROMIS (Prostate MR Imaging Study), which evaluated the diagnostic accuracy of mpMRI before biopsy and concluded that mpMRI might allow 27% of patients with raised prostate-specific antigen (PSA) to avoid biopsy.

Evaluation of Renal Masses

As detection rates of renal masses continue to increase, clinicians have aimed to improve characterisation of these lesions. The first step is to differentiate benign cysts from solid masses, which contain little or no fluid. This can generally be done with ultrasound, with indeterminate or solid masses then undergoing further characterisation with contrast-enhanced CT or MRI. The most common solid malignant renal masses are renal cell carcinoma and urothelial carcinoma, whereas the most common solid benign renal masses are angiomyolipoma (AML) and oncocytoma.

Magnetic resonance imaging is a useful imaging tool for diagnosis and characterisation of renal lesions because it provides excellent soft-tissue contrast. In renal cell carcinoma, a hypointense pseudo capsule may be seen on both T1 and T2-weighted images. Interruption of this capsule correlates with invasion of perirenal fat. DWI and dynamic contrast enhanced (DCE) can provide further information regarding the tumour histology: there appears to be an inverse relationship between the apparent diffusion coefficient (ADC) value and Fuhrman grade. MRI is thus useful in differentiating benign from malignant lesions as well as predicting the subtype and tumour grade.

Classic angiomyolipomas (AMLs) are identified on MRI because they manifest with the hallmark of bulk fat, providing a high T1 signal. Lipid-poor AMLs are more difficult to distinguish from renal cell carcinoma (RCC). The typical enhancement pattern is of early intense enhancement with subsequent washout, high signal-intensity index, and low tumour-to-spleen signal-intensity ratio.

Staging Investigations

MRI is utilised in the staging of many urological cancers, according to the tumour/node/metastases (TNM) classification.

In prostate cancer, T2WI is fundamental in assessing extra-capsular extension, seminal vesicle invasion, and lymph node metastasis. Staging accuracy is enhanced using endorectal surface coil and the evolving role of DWI and DCE.

MRI is increasingly used in the staging of bladder cancer to assist in the differentiation of T2 and T3 disease, having been demonstrated to better assess intramural and extravesicular tumour invasion compared with CT. High resolution T2WI of the bladder in three planes with a small field of view and large matrix are used to evaluate the detrusor muscle. Potential artefacts include inappropriate bladder distension, chemical shift, and motion artefact. Optimal bladder distension is achieved by having the patient void two hours before imaging. Bowel peristalsis can be minimised by administrating anti-motility agents. Chemical shift is reduced by increasing the bandwidth and selecting the frequency-encoding gradient direction that least interferes with examination of the bladder wall.

Staging of penile cancer can be improved with MRI in combination with induced erection using prostaglandin E1, to exclude tumour invasion of the corpora cavernosa. However, imaging is not a reliable tool for detecting abnormal inguinal nodes. Distant metastases are generally assessed using computerized tomography/proton emission tomography (CT/PET).

Advantages and Disadvantages

MRI has the obvious advantage of not using ionising radiation. It provides excelled contrast between different soft tissues and higher resolution than CT. It can also scan in any plane. However, machines remain significantly more expensive and scans take more time than CT. More artefacts are encountered in MRI. In addition, MRI is contraindicated in patients with internal ferrous objects, such as aneurysm clips. In children, a general anaesthetic may be required. It is also less useful in patients with claustrophobia, due to the enclosed space.

Further Reading

Payne, S. and Eardley, I. (2012). *Imaging and Technology in Urology: Principles and Clinical Applications*. New York: Springer.
Tublin, M.E. and Nelson, J. (2018). *Imaging in Urology*. New York: Elsevier.

Index

Page locators in **bold** indicate tables. Page locators in *italics* indicate figures. This index uses letter-by-letter alphabetization.

Ambulatory Urology and Urogynaecology, First Edition. Edited by Abhay Rane and Ajay Rane.
© 2021 John Wiley & Sons Ltd. Published 2021 by John Wiley & Sons Ltd.